The

FAST

LOW-CARB

KICKSTART

Plan

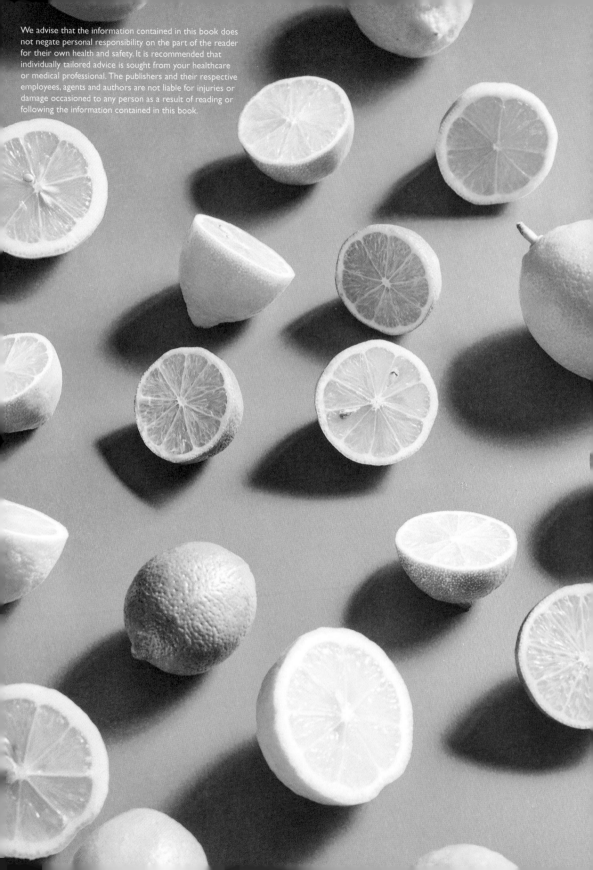

The FAST LOW-CARB KICKSTART Plan

The ultimate guide to intermittent fasting and low-carb eating for weight loss

LUKE HINES

plum. Pan Macmillan Australia

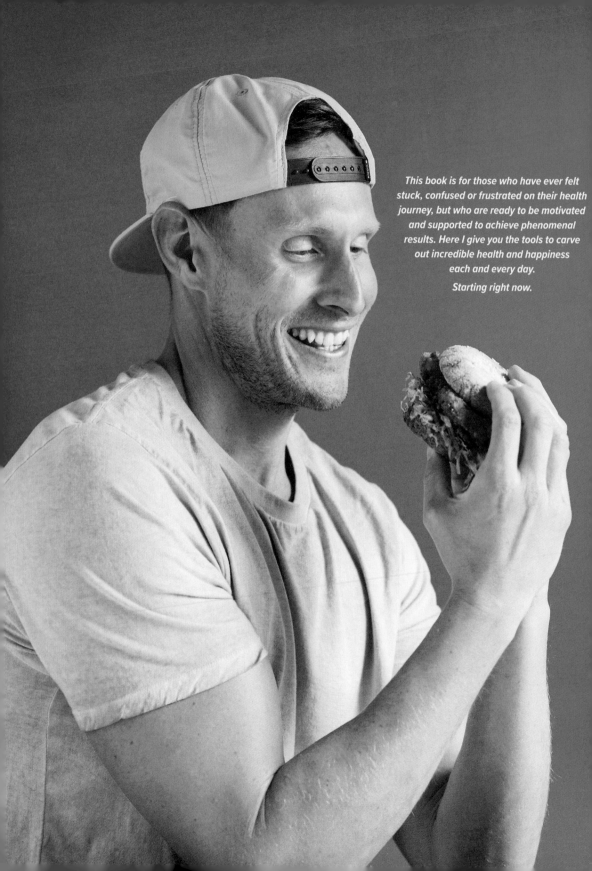

This book is for those who have ever felt stuck, confused or frustrated on their health journey, but who are ready to be motivated and supported to achieve phenomenal results. Here I give you the tools to carve out incredible health and happiness each and every day.

Starting right now.

CONTENTS

INTRODUCTION

As a nutritional therapist, personal trainer and passionate healthy cook, I have seen firsthand the profound positive effects that improving someone's health can have on their wellbeing. It is literally life changing.

When we lose excess body fat, increase healthy lean muscle mass, celebrate nutrient-dense real food and move daily we feel exponentially happier, sleep better and have increased energy and clarity, allowing us to live life to the full.

This is where *The Fast Low-Carb Kickstart Plan* comes in.

By combining the benefits of intermittent fasting with low-carb eating, this kickstart plan really works from the inside out. Because, when these scientifically and clinically proven methods of transforming your health are brought together, we end up with a really efficient, enhanced and time-effective approach to long-term wellness.

There is incredible hype surrounding all things related to low-carb, keto and fasting diets at the moment, with people experiencing many positive results. I put this book together to cut through all the noise with a really clear, succinct approach that absolutely anyone can implement.

In this book, you'll find all you the tools you need to make fast, realistic and lasting changes that you can implement for the rest of your life. The information packed into the following chapters reveals how intermittent fasting works while also giving you all the knowledge you need about going low carb, with over 70 delicious recipes to get you started. You'll be armed with the most up-to-date information on the impact that what we eat and when we eat it have on our overall wellbeing, plus you'll get all the tips, tricks and recipes you need to make real change happen, starting right now.

And while my kickstart is fantastic for anyone new to this approach, it's just as beneficial for seasoned fasters and low-carbers who simply need a reboot, refresh and reset.

Look, I get it. I know that overhauling your health can feel daunting. But please know it is easier, more delicious and less restrictive than you think. Fasting doesn't mean you can't eat, it's just about being mindful of when you eat. And going low carb doesn't mean you have to count calories, cut out entire food groups and miss out on the things you love – instead you'll be eating better, more nutritious and delicious food than ever before.

So, if you like the sound of …

- losing weight and keeping it off
- counting nutrients not calories
- no reduction of portions or skimping on flavour
- reducing your risk of chronic disease and inflammation
- a meal plan with 70+ low-carb recipes
- a four-week kickstart plan to get you on track
- a fad-free approach to long-term health
- tapping into your fat-burning potential
- implementing a potent, flexible and user-friendly approach to health
- discovering the motivation to stick to this long term

… then this book is for you!

I am not here to fill you with hope of unattainable results, or to set you up on a fad diet you simply cannot sustain in the real world. Instead this is a tried-and-tested plan for enhancing your wellbeing, both physically and mentally. For building a stronger, more resilient you.

Now, it's time to break things down further and delve into this exciting guide. But before we do, know this. Anything is possible when you're armed with the right knowledge and the motivation to make long-term change. You can do it and it will be incredible.

So what are you waiting for? Let's do this!

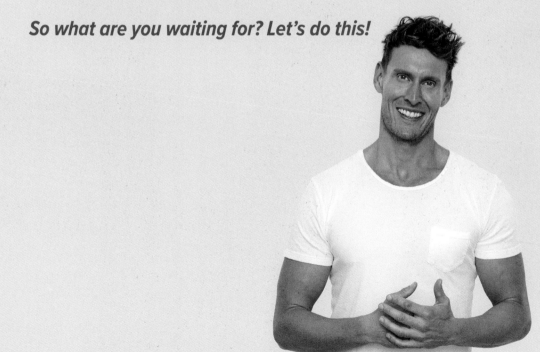

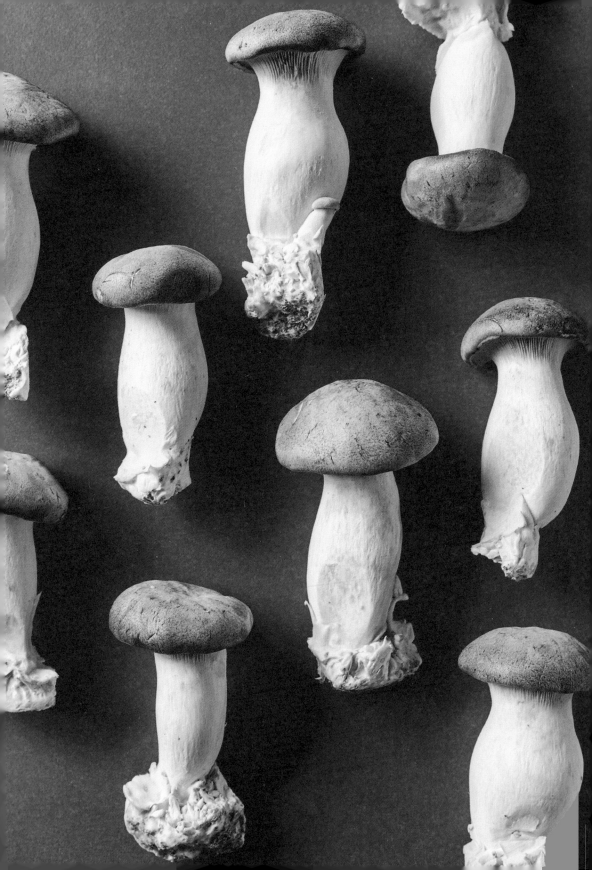

WHAT IS THE FAST LOW-CARB KICKSTART PLAN?

There is no doubting the incredible health benefits of intermittent fasting. As you'll discover in this book, limiting the window in which we eat has a profound effect on our bodies inside and out. Equally, following a low-carb or keto diet can very quickly and effectively produce results that benefit our overall health and wellbeing.

When you combine intermittent fasting with a low-carb diet, the results are exceptional. This should come as no surprise because the benefits of both consistently overlap, so it is something of a no-brainer that one supports the other.

Put simply, *The Fast Low-Carb Kickstart Plan* is a lifestyle program providing you with all the tools, tips and techniques – plus delicious recipes and motivation – necessary to make incredible long-term change when it comes to your health and happiness.

I'll educate you on the key factors and science behind intermittent fasting and how to follow a lower-carbohydrate approach, and then provide you with meal plans that accompany a four-week kickstart, helping you to implement this knowledge into practical, everyday use.

IT'S ABOUT THE MEALS, MINDSET AND MOVES

Now, although I talk predominately in this book about what and when to eat, for any health transformation to be successful we need to adopt a holistic approach to finding synergy between our Meals, Mindset and Moves.

What does that mean? Well, first and foremost it means celebrating nutrient-dense real food and ditching foods that can cause us harm or inflammation. Terms like 'dirty keto' or 'if it fits your macros' suggest that, as long as the macronutrient content of a food matches up to your daily requirements, you can eat whatever you want – including junk food. This couldn't be further from the truth. We need to source our macro and micronutrients from high-quality sources that provide our cells with energy in order to make every meal count, as they are an investment in our long-term health.

It also means that it is all well and good following this kickstart program as written, but to implement it successfully you need to align it with positive mindset techniques that will support you mentally on the journey. This means making sure that little voice inside your head 'backs' you and speaks positively about what you're doing. It's about being your biggest cheerleader and not your worst critic at a time when you may experience ups and downs, both mentally and physically.

Lastly, it means that we can eat all the healthy food in the world and work on cultivating a positive mindset, but unless we use the gift of our body we simply won't reach our full potential. So, find a way to move each and every day that you actually look forward to. For me this is the gym – working out helps me switch off and the endorphins it releases are really good for my mental wellbeing. But for you it might be a walk in the park, a jog on the beach, or kicking the footy with your friends or family. The key is to move your body so that you increase your agility, longevity, strength and stamina.

WHY DOES THE FAST LOW-CARB KICKSTART WORK?

Motivation can come and go, but what measures a plan's level of success is our ability to follow and maintain the approach for long-term weight loss, weight management and its overall positive impact on wellbeing – regardless of life's ups and downs.

The Fast Low-Carb Kickstart Plan works because it is a flexible lifestyle approach, not a diet based around calorie restriction or deprivation.

You get to eat what you want and how much you want, just as long as you follow the simple guidelines around the recommended eating window and embrace nutrient-dense, real ingredients.

It's a program that you can make work for you – around your lifestyle, schedule, preferred tastes and favourite foods. And this makes it much easier to stick to.

HOW OFTEN SHOULD I USE THE KICKSTART?

My advice is to start with the first four weeks of guided support contained in this book and then continue at your leisure. It really is up to you how often you implement intermittent fasting with a low-carbohydrate approach.

I have designed this program to start steady and build up to a longer fast. You'll find this beneficial from a lifestyle and sustainability perspective as you won't be going from zero to ten overnight. And although in my four-week plan I give some timing advice, it doesn't have to be too rigid – simply adjust your eating to fit in with your lifestyle around such factors as your work schedule, family events and special occasions.

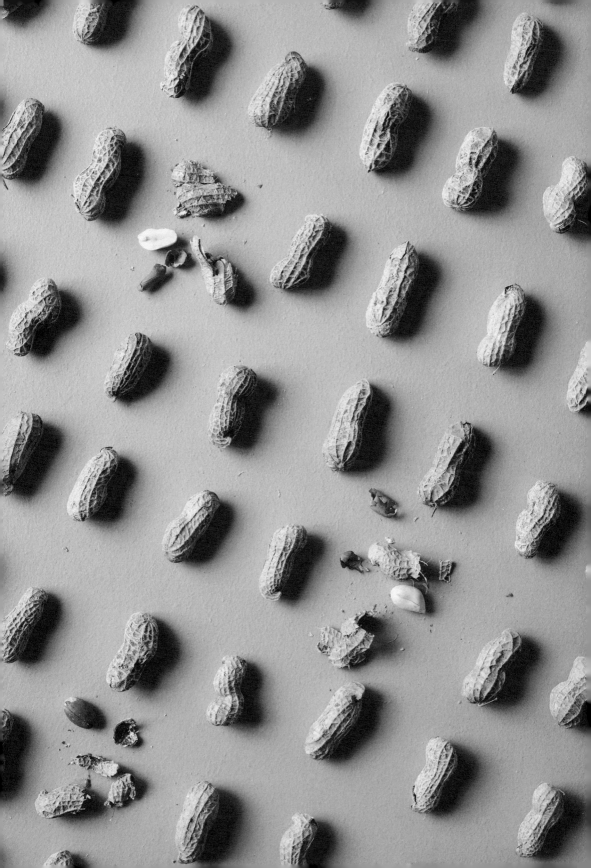

THE FOOD

Do you like the idea of cooking and eating foods that are filled with incredible flavour? Of following recipes that are as good for you as they are delicious, without ever feeling like you're on a diet or missing out on your favourite types of foods? Well then, my version of low-carb eating is for you.

Those of you familiar with my previous books will already know what I am about to say is true, but just to clarify for those who might just be joining me on their wellness journey: healthy food should never be boring, bland or dull. Instead it should always be filled with colour, flavour, nutrients and love.

I've said it before and I'll say it again – the key to long-term health success is being equipped with recipes that are enjoyable to make and a dream to eat for you, as well as your friends and family.

This book features some of my favourite low-carb recipes that are ideally suited to accompanying you during this kickstart. You'll learn more about how the fasting component works shortly, but right now I want to make sure you're well versed in all things low carb so you know what to cook and why.

WHAT IS A LOW-CARB DIET?

Like fasting, going low carb isn't anything new. First documented in the early 1900s, some doctors reduced carbohydrates and increased healthy fats as a way to treat patients with type I diabetes.

Going low carb means that we eat fewer carbohydrates and a higher proportion of fat. This way of eating is also sometimes referred to as 'low carb, healthy fat' (LCHF). When we avoid processed and refined sugars and starches our blood sugar tends to stabilise and the levels of the fat-storing hormone insulin drop. This increases the amount of fat we burn and makes us feel more satiated, reducing food intake and causing sustainable weight loss. Studies show that a low-carb approach can make it easier for us to lose weight, control our blood sugar, increase mental clarity and feel more energised.

When following my kickstart plan, you'll be consuming between 50 and 100 grams of carbohydrates per day. This level of carbohydrate intake promotes steady, sustainable and gradual weight loss. This is the sweet spot for many and is certainly my favourite way to live without ever feeling like I am on a diet. You'll get to enjoy a wide array of foods while still losing excess body fat, maintaining lean muscle mass and feeling fantastic. Studies have shown this to be a more sustainable long-term approach than a stricter keto diet for those of us who live busy lives.

THE ULTIMATE LOW-CARB FOOD PYRAMID

This pyramid is a great, easy-to-understand guide to the foods I love to celebrate as part of the kickstart plan.

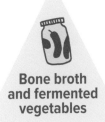

Bone broth and fermented vegetables

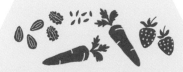

Below-ground vegetables, nuts, seeds and low-fructose fruits

Above-ground, non-starchy vegetables, herbs and spices

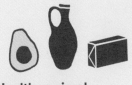

Healthy animal and plant-based fats

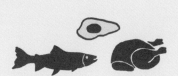

Well-sourced animal protein

GOING LOW CARB IN 3 SIMPLE STEPS

1. Remove refined carbs

Remove refined and processed sugars, packaged treats, grains and grain-based foods, including bread, rice and pasta from your diet. Instead you'll be sourcing your carbohydrates from real foods such as above-ground vegetables and low-fructose fruits. When it comes to celebrating the abundance of delicious above-ground vegetables, eat the rainbow, cook outside your comfort zone and use fresh herbs and spices as flavour enhancers.

↓

2. Increase healthy fats

Replace the carbohydrates you were eating with good-quality healthy fats in both wholefood form and oils. Eat fats in the form of free-range eggs, organic and pasture-fed meats, sustainable and wild-caught fish, avocados, nuts and seeds. Use avocado, hemp, macadamia and extra-virgin olive oil in your dressings and sauces, and elevate your food by baking, frying and barbecuing with extra-virgin coconut oil, grass-fed butter and ghee.

↓

3. Perfect your protein

Protein is a really important building block when it comes to dietary health and wellness. It helps regulate the body and repairs, builds and strengthens it while also keeping us satiated. Because this kickstart plan celebrates healthy fats in abundance, there is no need to focus on lean cuts of meat – instead you can enjoy the tastier, fattier cuts, such as free-range bacon, chicken thighs and omega-3-rich salmon. For anyone following a plant-based approach, be sure to supplement with plant-based protein sources that suit you.

Here is your daily intake of the three key macro-nutrients on a plate:

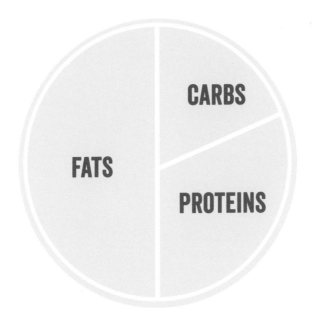

BUT WHAT ABOUT KETO?

Our bodies have two primary sources of fuel to choose from – glucose and fat. When we eat a diet high in carbs, we convert them into glucose and that is the fuel used to provide our bodies with the energy needed to function. When we significantly reduce our intake of carbohydrates, our body switches over to fat as its preferred fuel source. Ketosis, or 'going keto', is when the body enters a state where fat is its main fuel, with the fatty acids ingested supplying the body with ketones (by-products of the breakdown of fatty acids), which are used as its primary energy source. It can be harder to maintain a state of ketosis in the long term compared with a standard low-carb approach. That said, this kickstart can be done while following a strictly keto diet, so simply be mindful of your daily total carb intake. To remain in ketosis, you need to limit your intake to 20–50 grams of carbs per day.

YOUR FAST LOW-CARB KICKSTART KITCHEN

It is a good idea to prepare your kitchen by cleaning out your fridge, freezer and pantry. Donate or gift the foods you feel could derail your progress and stock up on the healthy staples listed below. Ingredients marked with an asterisk are fine only when consumed in moderation as per the recipe. If eaten in larger quantities, these foods can throw you out of the low-carb zone, so be mindful when consuming them for best results on your kickstart.

FRESH PRODUCE

- ARTICHOKE
- ASPARAGUS
- AVOCADOS
- BANANAS*
- BEETROOT*
- BLACKBERRIES
- BLUEBERRIES
- BOK CHOY
- BROCCOLI/BROCCOLINI
- BRUSSELS SPROUTS
- CABBAGE
- CAPSICUM
- CARROTS*
- CAULIFLOWER
- CELERY
- CHARD
- CHICORY GREENS
- CHILLIES
- CITRUS
- CORNICHONS
- CUCUMBER
- DAIKON
- EGGPLANT
- ENDIVE
- FENNEL
- GARLIC
- GINGER
- GREEN APPLES*
- GREEN PAPAYA
- HERBS
- KALE
- LEEKS
- LEMONGRASS
- MIXED LETTUCE
- MUSHROOMS
- OLIVES
- ONIONS
- PALM HEARTS*
- PARSNIPS*
- PUMPKIN
- RADICCHIO
- RADISHES
- RASPBERRIES
- ROCKET
- SPINACH
- SPRING ONION
- SQUASH
- STRAWBERRIES
- SWEET POTATOES*
- TOMATOES
- TURMERIC
- ZUCCHINI

FRIDGE

- BONE BROTH
- COCONUT AMINOS*
- ETHICAL AND SUSTAINABLE FISH AND SEAFOOD
- FILTERED WATER
- FREE-RANGE EGGS
- FREE-RANGE POULTRY, PORK AND GAME
- GRASS-FED BEEF
- MAYONNAISE/AIOLI
- MUSTARD
- NUT AND SEED MILKS: ALMOND, COCONUT AND HEMP
- PASTURED LAMB
- SAUERKRAUT
- SUGAR-FREE FISH SAUCE
- SUGAR-FREE TABASCO SAUCE
- SUGAR-FREE TOMATO SAUCE
- TAMARI
- TAMARIND PASTE
- UNSWEETENED COCONUT YOGHURT
- UNSWEETENED GHERKINS
- WELL-SOURCED OFFAL

FREEZER

- BONES FOR MAKING BROTH/STOCK
- BULK COOKED MEALS
- BULK SNACKS AND SLABS, SEE PAGE 176
- FROZEN BERRIES
- ICE FOR SMOOTHIES AND SMOOTHIE BOWLS, SEE PAGE 42
- LEFTOVER MEALS

PANTRY

- ALMOND MEAL
- APPLE CIDER VINEGAR
- CANNED COCONUT CREAM AND MILK
- CANNED YOUNG JACKFRUIT
- COCONUT: SHREDDED, DESICCATED AND FLAKED
- COCONUT BUTTER
- COCONUT FLOUR
- CURRY POWDER
- DRIED HERBS AND SPICES
- ESSENTIAL OILS: PEPPERMINT
- ETHICAL AND SUSTAINABLE CANNED FISH AND SEAFOOD
- FREEZE-DRIED BERRIES AND BERRY POWDER
- GLUTEN-FREE BAKING POWDER
- GRASS-FED GELATINE AND COLLAGEN POWDER
- MCT OIL/MCT KETO TONIC
- NUT BUTTERS: PEANUT, MACADAMIA, HAZELNUT ETC.
- NUTRITIONAL YEAST
- NUTS AND SEEDS
- ORGANIC COFFEE
- RAW CACAO BUTTER, NIBS AND POWDER
- SEA SALT AND CRACKED BLACK PEPPER
- SEED BUTTERS, TAHINI
- SUGAR-FREE CURRY PASTE
- TAPIOCA/ARROWROOT FLOUR*
- TOMATO PASTE AND PASSATA
- VANILLA BEAN: EXTRACT, POWDER AND PODS

HEALTHY COOKING FATS AND OILS

- COLD-PRESSED AVOCADO OIL
- COLD-PRESSED MACADAMIA OIL
- DUCK FAT
- EXTRA-VIRGIN COCONUT OIL
- EXTRA-VIRGIN OLIVE OIL
- GRASS-FED BUTTER
- GRASS-FED GHEE
- HEMP SEED OIL
- LARD
- TALLOW

SWEETENERS

- COCONUT SUGAR*
- GREEN LEAF STEVIA
- MONK FRUIT SWEETENER
- PURE MAPLE SYRUP*
- RAW HONEY*

YOUR SWEET SWEET GUIDE TO SWEETENERS

As you guys know I love a sweet treat, and I have designed the recipes in this book to support you on your low-carb journey. All the ingredients in my recipes will help you stay on track. In this book I use a number of my favourite sweeteners and you can choose the one that best fits with your personal plan. There are some that contain a moderate amount of carbohydrates and these can be used mindfully if you are taking a low-carb approach, and others that contain low to no carbohydrates and don't spike your blood sugar levels in any way, so these are great if you're sticking to a keto or very low-carb approach.

Monk fruit sweetener (syrup and granules)

Monk fruit sweetener is made from a fruit resembling a small green melon. The sweetness comes from naturally occurring chemical compounds known as mogrosides. These are extracted and turned into either 100% powdered monk fruit or pure monk fruit syrup. It has no effect on blood sugar levels and is extremely sweet. It has a slight aftertaste and only needs to be used in very small quantities. While 100% pure monk fruit sweetener is available, I prefer a blend of monk fruit and erythritol, which is a sugar alcohol that has no effect on blood sugar. I think this blend tastes better in sweet treats.

Green leaf stevia

Commonly known as the 'sugar leaf', stevia is a herb with a leaf that is 200–300 times sweeter than sugar. It contains no calories and is available in liquid, powder and tablets. Some brands add other artificial sweeteners so make sure you check the ingredients when purchasing. You only need to use a tiny amount and some brands can leave a slightly bitter aftertaste, so try a few and see which one you prefer.

Freeze-dried berries

Berries are the most nutritious and lowest in starchy carbs of all fruits. You can find freeze-dried berries and berry powders without additives in good health food stores. They make a fantastic sweetener in smoothies, raw desserts and baked goods and they add beautiful flavour to dishes. When used to decorate desserts, whole or crushed freeze-dried berries look spectacular. Freeze-dried raspberries are my favourite.

Coconut sugar

Coconut sugar comes from coconut palm blossom. It has a slightly caramel taste and smell, making it a fantastic ingredient for baking. It is rich in minerals such as magnesium, potassium and zinc, and its sugar content is made up mostly of sucrose, which is half fructose and half glucose. When looking for a healthy sweetener this is important because the lower the fructose content the better, as excessive consumption of fructose can be addictive and lead to hormonal imbalance.

Pure maple syrup

Pure maple syrup is made from evaporated maple tree sap. It is high in magnesium and zinc, which is important for immune system function, and is rich in calcium, B vitamins and antioxidants. Some might be surprised that I recommend maple syrup in low-carb recipes, but when used in small amounts it is a good sugar alternative. Enjoy it in moderation.

Raw honey

Unfiltered raw honey is one of the most nutrient dense of natural sweeteners. It is different from the types usually found in supermarkets. In conventional processing many of the essential nutrients are destroyed during pasteurisation and heating, so it is worth making the extra effort to find it in its most natural state. The glycaemic index rating of honey can vary depending on the botanical source – different blossoms make honey of varying sweetness. Because it is relatively high in carbohydrates, I recommend using honey in moderation when following my kickstart plan.

So what do I use in this book?

When monk fruit is listed in the recipes, I've used Lakanto monk fruit sweetener, which is a blend of monk fruit and erythritol. I find this works best as a syrup, but it can also be found in granules and used in the same quantities as the syrup. It is available from health food stores, some supermarkets and online, but if you can't source it, please use the chart below for the best alternatives.

HEALTHY SUGAR CONVERSION CHART

Use this chart to help you substitute sugar for other healthier sweeteners.

	LOW CARB			MODERATE CARB			
	100% monk fruit	Monk fruit sweetener blend	Green leaf stevia	Freeze-dried berries	Coconut sugar	Maple syrup	Raw honey
	0 g net carbs/ tablespoon	0 g net carbs/ tablespoon	6 g net carbs/ tablespoon	11 g net carbs/ tablespoon	11 g net carbs/ tablespoon	13.4 g net carbs/ tablespoon	17.3 g net carbs/ tablespoon
1 CUP SUGAR	1 teaspoon	1 cup	1 teaspoon	½ cup	½ cup	¾ cup	¾ cup

LOW-CARB KITCHEN SWAPS

Now that you know what going low carb entails and the abundance of deliciousness we have in store, let's take a look at some simple kitchen swaps that will help to make this transition even easier.

Hot chips and french fries → **Parsnip fries or Baked Butternut Fries (see page 86)**

Potato chips and processed snacks → **Crispy kale chips or seed crackers**

Soy sauce and teriyaki sauce → **Coconut aminos or tamari**

Wheat flour and rice flour → **Almond meal or coconut flour**

Pasta → **Spiralised zucchini or konjac noodles**

Rice → **Broccoli or Cauliflower Rice (see page 107)**

Tacos and tortillas → **Lettuce cups or Coconut Tortillas (see page 111)**

Mashed potatoes → **Cauliflower or pumpkin puree**

Bread and bread rolls	→	**Seeded Cauliflower Loaf (see page 54), Brilliant Bread (see page 56) or Bangin' Buns (see page 57)**
Dairy and soy milk	→	**Almond, coconut or hemp milk**
Burger buns	→	**Portobello mushrooms, lettuce cups or Bangin' Buns (see page 57)**
Refined seed oils	→	**Coconut, extra-virgin olive, hemp, macadamia or avocado oils**
Refined and processed sugary chocolate	→	**Luke's Block of Choc (see page 158)**
Milky sugary coffee	→	**MCT Power Up Coffee (see page 42)**
Alcohol	→	**Sparkling water with fresh lime or apple cider vinegar**

THE FAST

As you know, my kickstart plan is a two-pronged approach to wellness, where we combine the health benefits of a low-carb approach to eating and intermittent fasting to yield exceptional, lasting results. Now you know the basics behind going low carb, let's dive into fasting so we can put them together to create my structured four-week kickstart plan.

WHAT IS FASTING?

Fasting has been an integral part of many religions and cultures for centuries. While research is still in the early stages and has mostly been conducted on animals, fasting has been shown to have many possible health benefits, including the ability to help prolong life-span as well as the potential to inhibit the development of a range of illnesses and diseases, including cancer, diabetes and heart disease.

When we fast we allow our body to enter its optimal fat-burning zone – increasing our weight-loss potential by letting it tap into stored body fat as fuel. We also provide our body with the many health benefits that come from giving it a rest from constantly processing and digesting. Fasting increases energy, promotes cellular repair and autophagy (when your body consumes defective tissue in order to produce new cells), reduces insulin resistance and protects against type 2 diabetes, as well as lowering bad cholesterol and promoting overall longevity by keeping our mitochondria strong. In addition, fasting has proven positive outcomes when it comes to the brain, improving memory and helping to boost brain function, factors that may make it a helpful tool in the fight against neurodegenerative diseases such as Alzheimer's and Parkinson's.

Although there are many forms of fasting in the health space, there are two major approaches that are most commonly spoken about – full-day and part-day fasting.

Full-day fasting, also commonly referred to as the 5:2 approach, is when you eat just a quarter of your daily calories over a full day, but only on certain days of the week. When it comes to 5:2, it is five days of regular eating, with two days of restricted calorie intake.

Part-day fasting, also known as time-restricted eating or 16:8, is when you fast completely for a set number of hours each day, followed by a structured period of eating, or what I like to call nutrient-dense feasting. After your fast, rather than counting calories you can enjoy the many recipes in this book and all my others intuitively within your eating window, eating when you're hungry and stopping when you're full.

Full-day fast

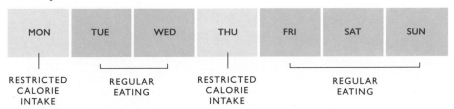

| MON | TUE | WED | THU | FRI | SAT | SUN |

RESTRICTED CALORIE INTAKE   REGULAR EATING   RESTRICTED CALORIE INTAKE   REGULAR EATING

Part-day fast

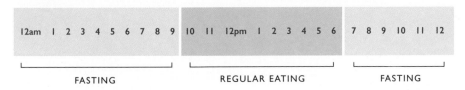

| 12am | 1 | 2 | 3 | 4 | 5 | 6 | 7 | 8 | 9 | 10 | 11 | 12pm | 1 | 2 | 3 | 4 | 5 | 6 | 7 | 8 | 9 | 10 | 11 | 12 |

FASTING   REGULAR EATING   FASTING

As you know, I am all about counting nutrients over calories and like to keep my recipes simple so the approach to fasting in this book is all about part-day fasting. Part-day fasting is great for those of us who might not be hungry at certain times of the day, live busy lifestyles with hectic schedules or lots of travel, keep physically active or need full mental focus and stamina, which can sometimes be difficult to achieve when following restricted calorie fasting.

The other reason I have structured this kickstart program around the part-day fasting approach is because it is generally a more sustainable and user-friendly method. Simply put, you fast for a certain number of hours (either 12, 16 or 18) each day and then follow my low-carb approach for the rest of the day (either 12, eight or six hours). This is how I fast because I don't need to worry about counting calories or minimising my portion sizes, and I don't feel deprived of good food when the realities of life happen. Let's take a closer look at how the different fasting windows work and which one might be right for you.

FASTING METHODS

Beginners – 12:12

The 12:12 fasting method is a great starting point for those completely new to this way of life. A good example would be fasting between 7 pm and 7 am. Interestingly enough, many of us may already be doing this – or close to it – but it's those late-night dinners and snacking during the evenings that trip us up. To begin tapping into our fat-burning zone, this 12-hour window of fasting is the perfect place to start. So take note of when you eat and increase the gap between those meals and you'll be achieving 12:12 in no time. This is the fast you will follow in week one of your kickstart plan.

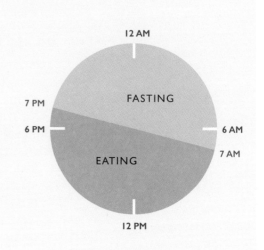

Intermediate – 16:8

The 16:8 fasting method is what I call the sweet spot when it comes to the various intermittent fasting options and is one that many people have success with. You'll fast for 16 hours over a 24-hour period and eat your nutrient-dense food in the eight-hour eating window. Considering most of your fasting is done while you're asleep, this yields great results in a really manageable way. I like to have my last meal at 6 pm and then wait until 10 am before breaking the fast. Start by pushing breakfast back a few hours, then eating an earlier dinner. This is the fast you will follow in weeks two and three of your program.

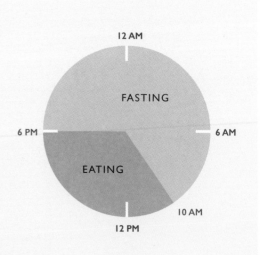

Advanced – 18:6

For serious weight-loss results, increase your fasting window to 18 hours, with a six-hour window of eating. So if your last meal is at 7 pm, don't break your fast until 1 pm. This can dramatically increase weight loss, but my advice is to first spend a decent period of time mastering the 12:12 and 16:8 fasting methods before advancing to this level. The biggest take away if you follow this regime is to make sure you meet all of your nutritional requirements in your six-hour eating window. So eat calorie-dense, nutrient-dense, varied foods for that much-needed diversity. This is the fast you will follow in week four of your kickstart.

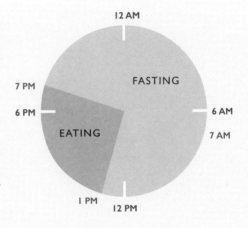

There are many diets and approaches to weight loss and long-term wellbeing where we can experience 'diet fatigue' – a period where our body adapts to the new regime, resulting in a plateau or reversal of our results, which in turn can reduce our motivation and increase the risk of falling back into old bad habits. The good news is that fasting makes it harder for the body to adapt as you are still eating a normal nutrient-dense diet when you do eat. Plus, the meal plans include loads of recipes that actually feel like treats, such as burgers, tacos and even fudge bites, that really satisfy your nutritional requirements. Because the food is so yum and the nutrients are so satiating, psychologically it is really easy to stick to, as you never feel like you're missing out.

HOW DOES IT WORK?

Many of us are used to eating for most of the day in some way. From the moment we wake when we eat breakfast, to the snacks we consume throughout the day, to late-night treats and nibbles. Research has shown this constant state of eating and digesting leads to weight gain, impairs the health of our cells and can accelerate the ageing process.

When we are fasting, we give our body a break from constantly processing food, presenting the energy powerhouses in our cells known as mitochondria with the opportunity to repair. We also allow our body to tap into an optimal fat-burning state.

Fasting has been shown to help:

- Reverse metabolic syndrome
- Manage obesity and weight loss
- Reduce blood pressure, improve cholesterol profiles and protect against heart disease
- Manage type 2 diabetes with significant reductions in insulin and blood glucose levels
- Improve brain health by producing BDNF (brain-derived neurotrophic factor) – a protein that stimulates the growth of new neurons and the connections between neurons
- Produce a compound that blocks part of the body's inflammatory process
- Give our gut bacteria a much-needed break, allowing us to restore normal levels of gut microbiota
- Beneficial bacterial colonies across the body to thrive and increase microbial diversity.

CHOOSING YOUR FASTING WINDOW

The good news about part-day fasting is that it is very versatile and adaptable to your lifestyle. It is up to you how you structure your eating windows, though I recommend you initially adjust and increase your non-eating windows by just two hours each day until you're at your desired fasting period.

If you're one of those people who naturally doesn't feel like breakfast, you are the perfect fit for 12 pm being the first meal of your day. Therefore, depending on whether your eating window is six or eight hours, you can enjoy all the deliciousness up until either 6 pm or 8 pm.

That said, many people are very physically or mentally active and require fuel upon (or close to) waking. If this is you, simply break your fast with your first meal at 8 am or 10 am and then restart your fasting period according to a 12:12, 16:8 or 18:6 fasting method.

Ultimately it is about structuring your meals around what is important to you and your lifestyle needs. You may prefer to skip breakfast, then break your fast with a decent brunch and enjoy a meal with your family. Or you may like to fuel-up in the morning before or after exercise and then recover with a big post-workout feed mid-morning without the need for a big meal later in the day. Look at your options and what fits with your life best, then set about making it work for you.

SO WHAT CAN I EAT?

Two of the questions I am most commonly asked are 'What am I allowed to have during my fasting period?' and, conversely, 'What can I eat in my eating window?'. Let's take a closer look.

WHAT CAN I HAVE WHEN I AM FASTING?

When you're fasting you are not allowed any food or drinks that contain calories. This is to prevent a spike in your blood glucose and insulin levels, which can throw you out of your fasting zone, increase cravings and decrease your fat-burning potential. This simple list is your basis for fasting-safe options.

- Filtered water, still or sparkling
- Black coffee
- Herbal tea
- Black tea

WHAT ABOUT MCT POWER UP COFFEE DURING MY FAST?

For fasting purists, consuming a single calorie technically breaks your fast. However, on my kickstart, there is a drink we can enjoy that means we don't completely restrict calories but still reap the benefits of intermittent fasting.

My MCT power up coffee (see page 42 for the recipe) is a combination of black coffee, grass-fed butter or ghee and MCT oil, a pure form of fat derived from coconut oil. Including this amazing drink in your meal plans is a game changer for those wanting to start and extend their intermittent fast.

The reason we can have this drink during our fast is because it contains fats only (no protein or carbs), meaning it won't interrupt autophagy and we'll stay in a fat-burning state. Fasting works because it keeps insulin levels low enough to keep your body in a fat-burning state. Fats from grass-fed butter or ghee and MCTs from coconut oil don't cause insulin levels to rise.

It is fantastic because after enjoying an MCT power up coffee our body will get the signal that we've eaten, and you won't feel hungry. Then, we can extend our intermittent fast a few hours longer for even more fat-burning benefits. The majority of benefits of intermittent fasting come from autophagy, so an extra hour or two makes a big difference.

WHAT CAN I HAVE WHEN I AM NOT FASTING?

By now, you should already know the good news – my kickstart plan allows you to celebrate nutrient-dense foods in abundance with no need to count calories and without feeling like you're restricting any of your favourite foods. For a detailed guide of what to eat and how to implement these fasting styles, check out the tailored weekly meal plans on the following pages.

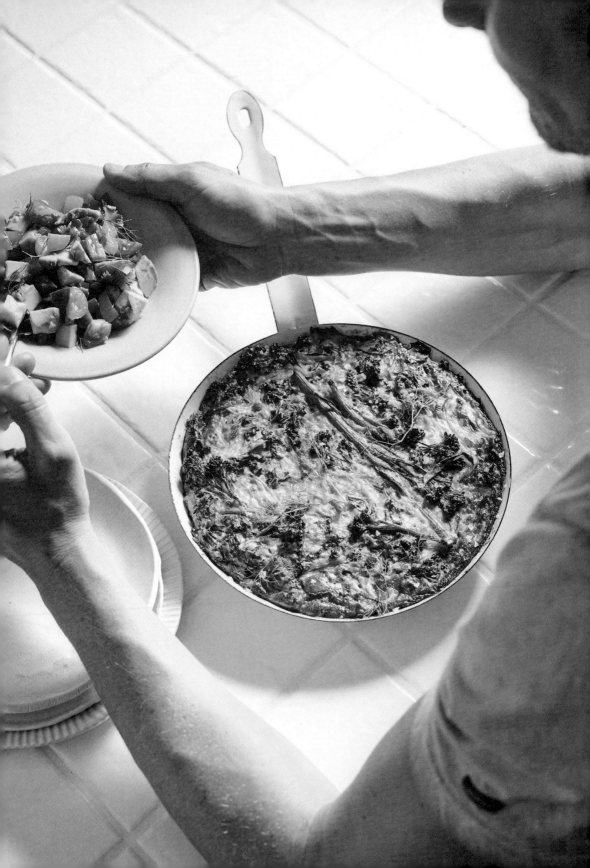

THE FOUR-WEEK KICKSTART AND MEAL PLANS

Now you are well versed in all things intermittent fasting and low-carb eating, let's dive into how to implement the kickstart. Over the following pages you'll see my four suggested weekly meal plans for the kickstart, which have been broken down as follows:

WEEK ONE – 12:12

Week one is structured around a 12:12 fasting window with a focus on the simplest and quickest recipes in the book. This is the perfect starting point, regardless of whether you're a beginner to the world of fasting and low-carb eating or not. It's a great chance to reset the body with real food and remind yourself what it is like to slightly stretch your eating window.

WEEK TWO – 16:8

This week we transition to a 16:8 structure with our fast, while the addition of some new recipes brings variety and nutrient diversity – the key to balanced health. You'll have to wait an extra two hours before your first meal, followed by a shorter, eight-hour eating window that ends two hours earlier than the previous week's.

WEEK THREE – 16:8

Week three really reinforces what you've done in week two. Being the sweet spot of fasts, it is helpful to really settle into this length of fast and master the eight-hour eating window before considering taking it to the next level. Feel free to swap out any of the recipes for some of your favourites from previous weeks, or cook in bulk to have extra on hand for the following days.

WEEK FOUR – 18:6

Week four gives you the opportunity to really enhance and amplify your results by adding an extra two hours to your total fast in any 24-hour period. Most people find 12 pm till 6 pm to be the ideal eating window. Please stay at 16:8 this week if you feel that is working for you and you're happy with the results so far – this next phase is absolutely optional, depending on how you're feeling, your lifestyle and your goals.

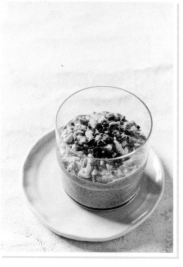

Choc Peanut Butter Pudding (page 44)

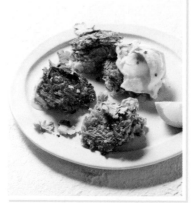

Pumpkin and Zucchini Bites with Poached Eggs and Avo (page 58)

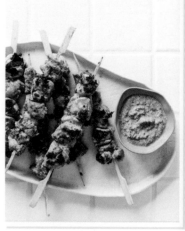

Charred Coconut Chicken Skewers (page 116)

WEEK ONE – 12:12

	DAY 1	DAY 2	DAY 3
MEAL 1	Creamy Hemp and Coconut Porridge (page 52)	Japanese Omelette (page 66)	Loaded Avocados with Lemony Dream Chee (page 72)
MEAL 2	Seeded Cauliflower Loaf (page 54) (with 2 eggs your way, nut butter, tinned fish or ½ avocado)	Leftover Crispy Butter Chicken Salad (page 114)	Leftover Spicy Pork Burgers with Macadam Harissa (page 140)
MEAL 3	Crispy Butter Chicken Salad (page 114) *(LND – Lunch Next Day)	Spicy Pork Burgers with Macadamia Harissa (page 140) *(LND)	Gorgeous Green Fish Parcels (page 100) *(LND)
SNACK	Phenomenal Fudge Bites (page 50)	Seeded Cauliflower Loaf (page 54) (with grass-fed butter or your favourite nut butter)	MCT Power Up Coffe (page 42)

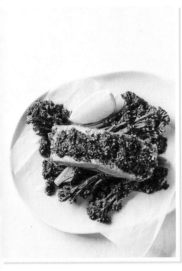

Gorgeous Green Fish Parcels (page 100)

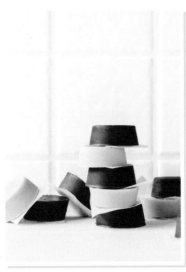

Phenomenal Fudge Bites (page 50)

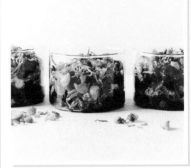

Apple and Berry Crumble Cups (page 172)

DAY 4	**DAY 5**	**DAY 6**	**DAY 7**
umpkin and Zucchini tes with Poached Eggs and Avo (page 58)	Choc Peanut Butter Pudding (page 44)	Seeded Cauliflower Loaf (page 54) (with 2 eggs your way, nut butter, tinned fish or ½ avocado)	Leftover Salmon and Pumpkin Fishcakes (page 98)
tover Gorgeous Green sh Parcels (page 100)	Leftover Charred Coconut Chicken Skewers (page 116)	Leftover Minute Steak and Buttery Mushrooms (page 148)	Baked Butternut Fries (page 86)
Charred Coconut Chicken Skewers (page 116) *(LND)	Minute Steak and Buttery Mushrooms (page 148) *(LND)	Salmon and Pumpkin Fishcakes (page 98) *(LND)	Mexican Meatballs with Salsa Sauce (page 144) *(LND)
Seeded Cauliflower Loaf (page 54) ith grass-fed butter or your favourite nut butter)	Phenomenal Fudge Bites (page 50)	MCT Power Up Coffee (page 42)	Apple and Berry Crumble Cups (page 172)

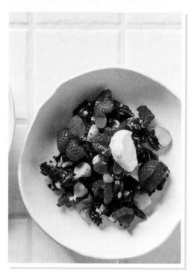

Chunky Granola Clusters (page 48)

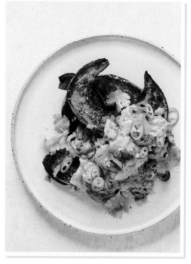

Curried Scramble with Pumpkin Wedges (page 68)

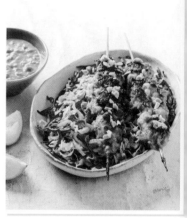

Simple Satay and Slaw (page 120)

WEEK TWO – 16:8

	DAY 1	DAY 2	DAY 3
MEAL 1	Spicy Brekkie Muffins (page 60)	Choc–Collagen Smoothie (page 42)	MCT Power Up Coffee (page 42)
MEAL 2/SNACK	Leftover Mexican Meatballs with Salsa Sauce (page 144)	Leftover Simple Satay and Slaw (page 120)	Chunky Granola Clusters (page 48)
MEAL 3	Simple Satay and Slaw (page 120) *(LND)	Bangin' Burgers with Mushroom Buns (page 150)	Barramundi Lettuce Cups (page 96)

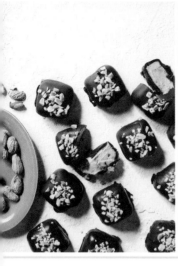

Simple 'Snickers' Bites (page 182)

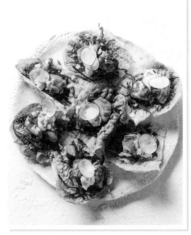

Barramundi Lettuce Cups (page 96)

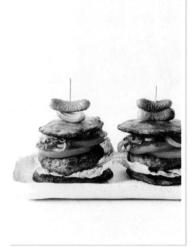

Bangin' Burgers with Mushroom Buns (page 150)

DAY 4	DAY 5	DAY 6	DAY 7
Chunky Granola Clusters (page 48)	Two-Minute Breakfast Eton Mess (page 46)	Curried Scramble with Pumpkin Wedges (page 68)	The Big Breakfast Plate (page 62)
Simple 'Snickers' Bites (page 182)	MCT Power Up Coffee (page 42)	Simple 'Snickers' Bites (page 182)	Green Apple Muffins (page 166)
Chicken 'n' Bacon Wraps with Zesty Avocado Smash (page 124)	Fiery Fish Curry with Cauliflower Rice (page 106)	Marinated Lamb Kofta with Terrific Turmeric Sauce (page 154) and Gorgeous Green Tabbouleh (page 78)	Ras-el-Hanout Chook with Chilli and Lime Yoghurt (page 122)

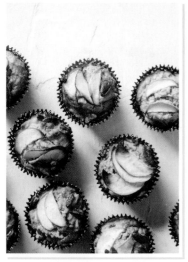

Green Apple Muffins (page 166)

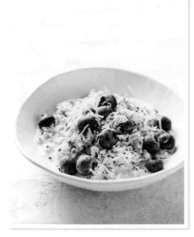

Creamy Hemp and Coconut Porridge (page 52)

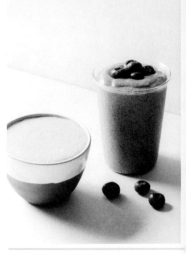

MCT Power Up Coffee (page 42)

WEEK THREE – 16:8

	DAY 1	DAY 2	DAY 3
MEAL 1	Green Apple Muffins (page 166)	Brilliant Bread (page 56) (with 2 eggs your way, nut butter, tinned fish or ½ avocado)	Choc–Collagen Smoo (page 42)
MEAL 2/SNACK	MCT Power Up Coffee (page 42)	Heavenly Hemp Slab (page 176)	MCT Power Up Coff (page 42)
MEAL 3	Leftover Ras-el-Hanout Chook with Chilli and Lime Yoghurt (page 122)	Jerk Drumsticks with Zesty Lime Cauliflower Smash (page 132)	Kaddo Bourani (page 146)

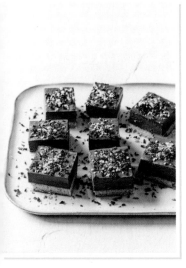

Heavenly Hemp Slab (page 176)

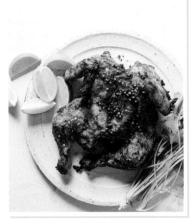

Ras-el-Hanout Chook with Chilli and Lime Yoghurt (page 122)

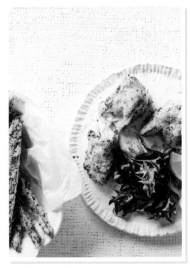

Herby Fried Fish and Chips (page 108)

DAY 4	**DAY 5**	**DAY 6**	**DAY 7**
⋯eftover Kaddo Bourani ⋯page 146) with Brilliant Bread (page 56)	Creamy Hemp and Coconut Porridge (page 52)	Veggie-loaded Mexican Frittata (page 64)	Brilliant Bread (page 56) (with 2 eggs your way, nut butter, tinned fish or ½ avocado)
Heavenly Hemp Slab (page 176)	MCT Power Up Coffee (page 42)	Heavenly Hemp Slab (page 176)	Mini Veggie Pies (page 90)
Chargrilled Pork Skewers with Tahini Dressing (page 138) and Sensational Sumac Steaks (page 84)	Chicken Curry Muffins (page 128) and Baby Spinach Salad with Minty Cashew Dressing (page 76)	Herby Fried Fish and Chips (page 108)	Luke's 'Zinger' Burger (page 126)

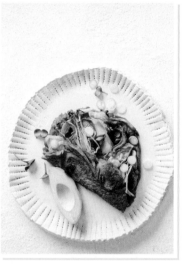

Japanese Omelette (page 66)

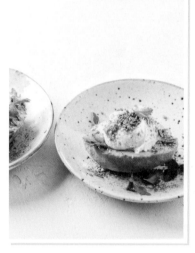

Loaded Avocados with Lemony Dream Cheese (page 72)

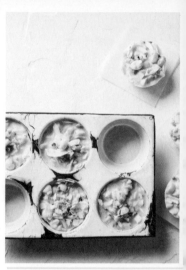

Macadamia Coconut Fat Bombs (page 178)

WEEK FOUR – 18:6

	DAY 1	DAY 2	DAY 3
MEAL 1	Japanese Omelette (page 66)	Bangin' Buns (page 57) (with 2 eggs your way, nut butter, tinned fish or ½ avocado)	Loaded Avocados with Lemony Dream Cheese (page 72)
MEAL 2/SNACK	MCT Power Up Coffee (page 42)	Macadamia Coconut Fat Bombs (page 178)	MCT Power Up Coffee (page 42)
MEAL 3	Chicken Mole (page 134)	Zingy Fish Tacos with Smashed Avo (page 110)	Crispy Cayenne Chicken with Simple Salsa (page 118)

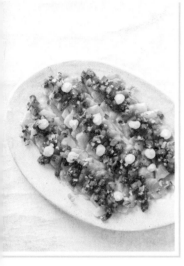

Simple Ceviche with Avocado Cream and Salsa (page 102)

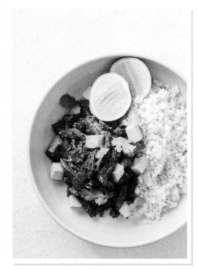

Chicken Mole (page 134)

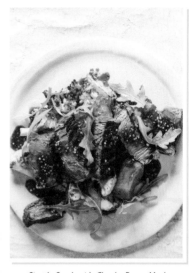

Simple Steak with Chunky Roast Mash (page 142)

DAY 4	DAY 5	DAY 6	DAY 7
Bangin' Buns (page 57) (with 2 eggs your way, nut butter, tinned fish or ½ avocado)	MCT Power Up Coffee (page 42)	Magnificent Mushroom Skewers (page 80)	MCT Power Up Coffee (page 42)
Macadamia Coconut Fat Bombs (page 178)	Macadamia Coconut Fat Bombs (page 178)	Peanut Butter Cream Cookies (page 174)	Simple Ceviche with Avocado Cream and Salsa (page 102)
Simple Steak with Chunky Roast Mash (page 142)	Chargrilled Zucchini with Avocado Hummus (page 82)	Spicy Coconut Fish Bites (page 104) with Raw Rainbow Ribbons (page 74)	Sri Lankan Lamb Curry Roast and Really Good Raita (page 152) with Spicy Broccoli Pakora (page 88)

WHAT'S NEXT?

After you've completed your initial four-week kickstart, continue this way of life as you please, choosing a 12:12, 16:8 or 18:6 fasting cycle, depending on your results and lifestyle. 12:12 is often for those who just want to maintain their current results, 16:8 is a fantastic, sustainable option for most people long-term, and 18:6 is excellent for those wanting to really enhance and amplify their results. Please remember that it takes about three to six weeks for the brain and body to adapt to fasting, so depending on how you respond, be patient and stick with it.

KICKSTART TIPS AND TRICKS

- Avoid refined, processed and packaged foods. Cooking from scratch is the key to avoiding hidden nasties.

- Drink water, then drink some more water. Consuming water during your fasts will help you feel full and hydrated.

- Be clear on your goals from the outset. Write them down and refer to them if you're experiencing a rough period during a fast.

- Schedule your fasting around life and social engagements. Don't let this way of life stop you hanging out with friends and family.

- If eating off plan, focus on filling your plate with colourful above-ground vegetables and healthy plant-based fats, as well as moderate serves of well-sourced protein, nuts, seeds and low-fructose fruit.

- Shop organic, local and as fresh as possible.

- Clean out your pantry, fridge and freezer to eliminate temptations.

- Avoid alcohol for a minimum of the initial four weeks of your kickstart. (As it is high in calories and not easily metabolised by the body, I don't see alcohol as playing a part in a long-term healthy lifestyle. It can lead to a lack of energy and poorer lifestyle choices, so the best advice, really, is to minimise your alcohol consumption.)

- Cook in bulk and stock the fridge with leftovers and meals that you can heat and eat so you've always got something healthy and low carb on hand.

- Drink bone broth – it is a game-changer that promotes good health – and eat fermented vegetables daily.

- Fast when you're distracted and busy – the time will pass much more quickly and you'll be feasting in no time.

- Plan your exercise and training around your eating windows, so you're energised and can enjoy food for recovery. (Some people report having extra energy to exercise when fasting. Everyone is different so just listen to your body and do what works for you.)

- Don't overeat during your eating window. Listen to your body, eat when hungry and stop when full. Don't just eat for the sake of it or your excess calorie intake may outweigh the benefit of your fast.

- Make an MCT power up coffee (see page 42) if you're fading and need some serious help during a long fast.

- Avoid fasting if you're pregnant or breastfeeding.

- Fasting is not recommended for anyone under 18, people who are underweight or the elderly.

3, 2, 1, GO!

Now, before you jump right in, it's important to understand one thing. Life happens. There will be any number of things – including social events, special occasions, travel and work commitments – that can upset your new way of life. For long-term success, it is important that you are able to adapt when everyday life interferes with your best-laid plans.

If you get off-track or there is a moment when you cannot stick to the plan for whatever reason, the best thing to do is to simply dust yourself off and get back into it as soon as possible. Don't let what might feel like a bad day turn into a bad week, then month, then year. Small, incremental steps each day lead to long-term, sustainable and realistic change. The key is to keep going, regardless of the pace.

Many of you might be following this program to lose excess body fat – that is certainly one of the fantastic benefits, but don't get caught up in any stress around your weight, how fast you lose it or the number of calories you consume. This plan is designed to enable you to switch into a state of physical and mental wellbeing where your body works with ease, without the mental stressors often associated with a diet.

And it is important that I clarify that, although my kickstart plan benefits many people, it's not for everyone. Some individuals should seek advice from a health professional before changing their diet or lifestyle like this – this can come down to an unhealthy history with food, an ongoing medical condition, or individual health circumstances. Always make sure you have the right medical advice and support. And whoever you are, be sure to be kind to yourself, cook your heart out and – most of all – have fun.

Right. You can do this. Let's go!

BREAD

KFAST

MCT POWER UP COFFEE + CHOC-COLLAGEN SMOOTHIE

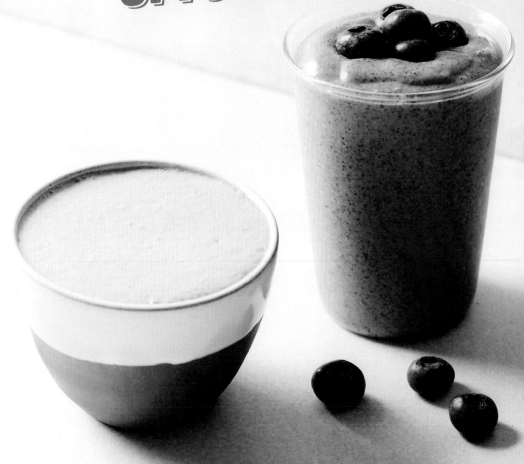

THIS IS HOW I ENJOY MY COFFEE EVERY SINGLE DAY, AND I SWEAR BY ITS INCREDIBLE HEALTH BENEFITS. IF INCREASED ENERGY, MOOD, FOCUS AND CLARITY ARE SOMETHING YOU'D LIKE, THEN LOOK NO FURTHER THAN THIS KILLER COMBINATION OF INGREDIENTS.

SERVES 1

250 ml (1 cup) freshly brewed
   black coffee
1 tablespoon MCT oil
1 teaspoon grass-fed butter or ghee

Put all the ingredients in a food processor and blitz until well combined, thick and frothy. Pour into your favourite mug, glass or re-usable coffee cup and enjoy.

GOOD TO KNOW: *The reason this drink works wonders is its combination of medium-chain triglycerides (MCTs) and a type of fat uniquely found in grass-fed butter and ghee. MCTs are a readily used source of energy that our body and mind thrives on, while grass-fed butter and ghee contains butyrate, a fatty acid that has been shown to help promote good gut health.*

HEALTH HACK: *Try adding some collagen powder and/or medicinal mushroom powder to this drink to increase its healing benefits.*

THOSE OF YOU WHO ARE FAMILIAR WITH MY RECIPES WILL KNOW THAT CHOCOLATE IS MY WEAKNESS. SO IT'LL COME AS NO SURPRISE THAT I PACKED THIS SMOOTHIE RECIPE FULL OF RAW CACAO, AND NOT JUST BECAUSE OF ITS INCREDIBLE HEALTH BENEFITS BUT BECAUSE … WELL, CHOCOLATE.

SERVES 1

125 ml (½ cup) coconut milk
125 ml (½ cup) filtered water
100 g (1 cup) fresh or frozen
   blueberries, plus extra to serve
2 tablespoons collagen powder
   (see Good to Know)
1 heaped tablespoon cacao powder
½ banana
½ avocado
1–2 drops of liquid stevia or
   1 tablespoon monk fruit syrup
   (optional)
½ teaspoon vanilla bean paste
   or powder
6 ice cubes

Blitz all the ingredients in a food processor or high-speed blender until smooth. Pour into a glass, add a few extra blueberries on top and drink up!

GOOD TO KNOW: *Collagen is a fantastic source of protein that can help to heal our gut, promote healthy skin, hair and nails, and support overall wellbeing. Collagen powders can be found at health food stores and online retailers – where they are available as flavoured blends or in natural and unsweetened form – and make an great alternative to whey-based protein powders.*

HEALTH HACK: *This smoothie is a fantastic example of how you can combine an excellent source of protein like collagen and small amounts of lower-fructose fruits such as blueberries and banana with larger amounts of healthy fats in the form of coconut milk and avocado to make a balanced low-carb meal.*

CHOC PEANUT BUTTER PUDDING

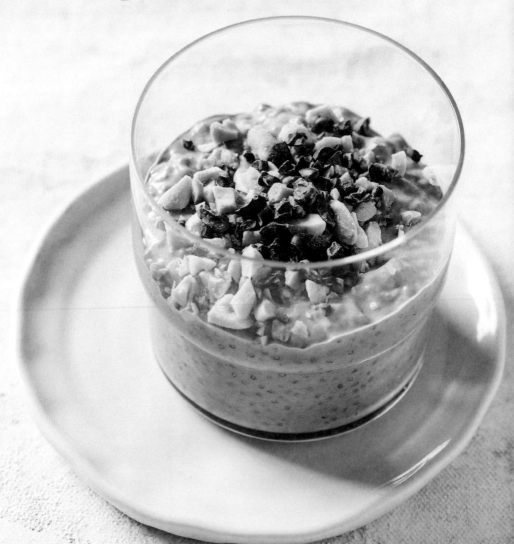

THIS LOVELY LITTLE CHIA PUDDING MAKES AN EXCELLENT BREKKIE, SNACK OR EVEN LUNCH ON THE RUN. IT'S A GREAT RECIPE TO LEARN OFF BY HEART AND MAKE IN BULK AT THE START OF A BUSY WEEK, SO YOU HAVE SOMETHING QUICK AND HEALTHY TO GRAB ON YOUR WAY OUT THE DOOR FOR THOSE DAYS WHEN TIME GETS AWAY FROM YOU.

SERVES 2

250 ml (1 cup) unsweetened almond, hemp or coconut milk

125 ml (½ cup) coconut milk

2 tablespoons cacao powder

½ teaspoon vanilla bean paste or powder

2–3 drops of liquid stevia or 2 tablespoons monk fruit syrup

3 tablespoons crunchy salted peanut butter, plus extra to serve

40 g (⅓ cup) white chia seeds

2 teaspoons cacao nibs

2 teaspoons roasted peanuts, roughly chopped

Place the milks, cacao powder, vanilla, sweetener of choice and peanut butter in a high-speed blender and blitz on high until smooth. Add the chia seeds and pulse a few times just to incorporate (you want to be careful not to blend too far as the chia seeds need to be left whole to do their thing), then transfer the mixture to a bowl, cover and place in the fridge for at least 1 hour, but preferably overnight. You want it to chill and thicken to a pudding-like consistency.

To serve, divide the pudding between two glasses and top with the cacao nibs, toasted peanuts and a little extra peanut butter.

GOOD TO KNOW: *If you'd like more of this recipe on hand for snacks and breakfast across the week, simply double or triple the quantities. Store in an airtight container in the fridge for up to 4 days. Top with the cacao nibs and peanuts just before serving.*

HEALTH HACK: *I love to use peanut butter in this recipe — it's low carb and really nutrient dense, which helps keep you feeling fuller for longer, plus it has a similar healthy fat ratio to olive oil, meaning it has many heart-healthy benefits.*

2-MINUTE BREAKFAST ETON MESS

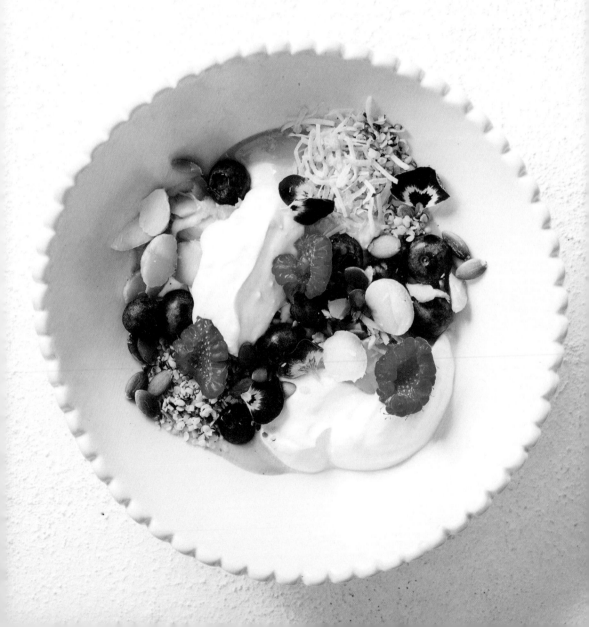

THIS IS A REALLY EASY TREAT TO THROW TOGETHER FOR THOSE MORNINGS WHEN YOU FIND YOURSELF SERIOUSLY SHORT OF TIME BUT STILL LOOKING FOR NOURISHMENT. PACKED WITH HEALTHY FATS AND NATURAL SWEETNESS, IT'S PERFECT FOR ANY TIME OF THE DAY.

SERVES 1

125 g (½ cup) coconut yoghurt or canned coconut cream
3 tablespoons blueberries, plus extra to serve
1 tablespoon peanut or macadamia butter
1 tablespoon MCT oil (optional)
1 tablespoon macadamia nuts, toasted and roughly chopped
1 tablespoon pumpkin seeds
2 teaspoons hulled hemp seeds (hearts)
1 tablespoon shredded coconut, toasted

TO SERVE
raspberries
edible flowers (optional)

Place the coconut yoghurt or cream, blueberries, peanut or macadamia butter and MCT oil, if using, in a serving bowl and use a spoon to swirl the ingredients together to create a lovely, colourful pattern.

Sprinkle over the macadamia nuts, pumpkin seeds, hemp seeds and flaked coconut and finish off with some extra blueberries, raspberries and edible flowers, if using. Serve immediately.

GOOD TO KNOW: *Coconut yoghurt works really well in this recipe because it holds its form when mixed with the other ingredients, plus it adds a lovely slightly tart taste compared to plain coconut cream.*

HEALTH HACK: *Frozen blueberries are just as good for you as fresh as no nutrients are lost in the freezing process. They are a great, cost-effective way of getting good-quality berries in your diet — just try to hunt down organic ones if you can so that you know they haven't been exposed to any nasties.*

CHUNKY GRANOLA CLUSTERS

SERVES 12

300 g (3 cups) pecans, roughly
   chopped
160 g (1 cup) macadamia nuts,
   roughly chopped
55 g (1 cup) flaked coconut
60 g (½ cup) pumpkin seeds
3 tablespoons cacao nibs
1 egg white, lightly beaten
2 tablespoons filtered water
3 tablespoons coconut oil, melted
60 g (½ cup) cacao powder
3 tablespoons collagen powder
   (optional)
125 g (½ cup) smooth peanut butter
1 teaspoon vanilla bean paste
   or powder
3 tablespoons monk fruit syrup, honey,
   maple syrup or coconut nectar

TO SERVE
raspberries, lightly mashed with a fork
coconut yoghurt
edible flowers (optional)

Preheat the oven to 180°C and line a baking tray with baking paper.

In a large bowl, combine the nuts, flaked coconut, pumpkin seeds and cacao nibs. Set aside.

In a small bowl, whisk the egg white and water until bubbly and slightly foamy. Add the coconut oil, cacao powder, collagen powder (if using), peanut butter, vanilla and sweetener of choice and whisk until well combined.

Pour the wet ingredients over the dry ingredients and stir everything well to combine.

Spread the mixture evenly across the prepared tray and bake for 35–40 minutes, rotating the tray halfway through cooking, until dry to the touch and crispy.

Remove the granola from the oven and leave to cool completely. Once cool, use a spatula to get under the granola and break it up into large clusters.

Serve topped with some raspberries, a dollop of coconut yoghurt and some edible flowers, if desired.

GOOD TO KNOW: *This delicious recipe can be made in bulk and stored in an airtight container in the pantry for up to 1 month.*

HEALTH HACK: *The reason I specifically celebrate pecans and macadamia nuts in this recipe is due to their wonderful omega-3 to omega-6 ratio, which makes them great sources of anti-inflammatory healthy fat.*

LET'S BE HONEST, WHEN IT COMES TO GRANOLA CHUNKS SIZE DOES MATTER, SO IF YOU LIKE YOURS BOTH GIANT AND DELICIOUS, THEN THIS INCREDIBLE RECIPE IS FOR YOU. SERVE IT UP WITH RASPBERRIES AND COCONUT YOGHURT LIKE THIS, OR SIMPLY GRAB A FEW CLUSTERS TO EAT ON THE GO.

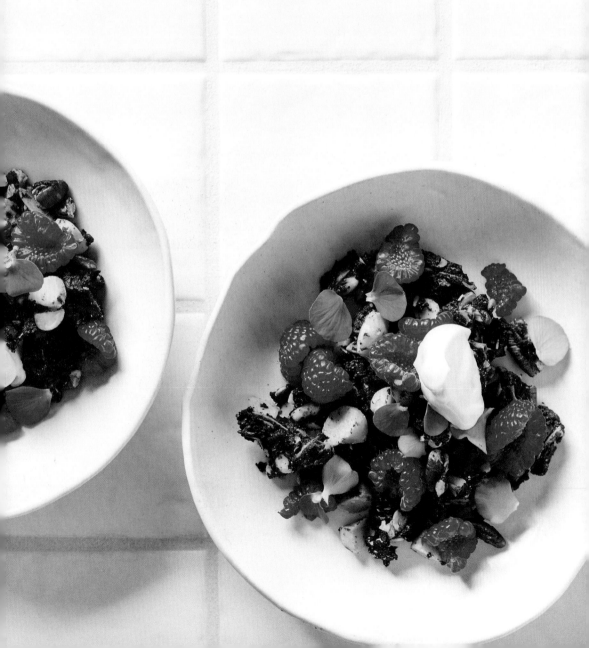

PHENOMENAL FUDGE BITES

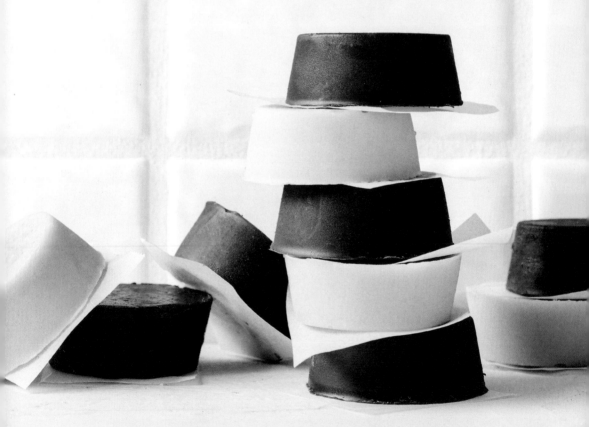

THESE AWESOME LITTLE FUDGE BITES MAKE A GREAT MORNING (OR ANYTIME) TREAT. INSPIRED BY MY LOVE OF 'TOP DECK' CHOCOLATE, I HAVE BROKEN THIS RECIPE DOWN INTO TWO VERSIONS — ONE DARK CHOCOLATE, ONE WHITE — SO THERE'S SOMETHING HERE TO SUIT ALL TASTE BUDS. FEEL FREE TO MAKE JUST ONE OR BOTH VERSIONS.

MAKES 12

DARK CHOCOLATE FUDGE
115 g (½ cup) cacao butter, melted
125 ml (½ cup) coconut oil, melted
250 g (1 cup) smooth peanut butter
125 g (1 cup) cacao powder
1 teaspoon vanilla bean paste
   or powder
2–4 drops of liquid stevia or 250 ml
   (1 cup) monk fruit syrup

WHITE CHOCOLATE FUDGE
115 g (½ cup) cacao butter, melted
125 ml (½ cup) coconut oil, melted
250 g (1 cup) macadamia butter
250 g (1 cup) coconut butter
1 teaspoon vanilla bean paste
   or powder
2–4 drops of liquid stevia or 250 ml
   (1 cup) monk fruit syrup

Line a 12-hole muffin tray with silicone moulds or paper cases.

Melt the cacao butter, coconut oil and peanut or macadamia butter together in a small saucepan over low heat, stirring, until thick and creamy.

Depending on whether you're making the dark or white chocolate fudge, add the remaining ingredients as listed and gently whisk until well combined.

Pour the mixture into the prepared muffin tray and transfer to the freezer for 30 minutes to chill and firm. The bites are now ready to eat or will keep in the fridge in an airtight container for up to 7 days.

GOOD TO KNOW: *Don't have a muffin tray or silicone moulds? Simply pour the fudge mixture into a small baking dish lined with baking paper, then chill in the freezer as above before cutting into squares.*

HEALTH HACK: *Arguably the peanut butter of the tropics, coconut butter is made by pureeing coconut flesh, including the oil. Solid at room temperature and softening when heated, the end result is a spread with a strong coconut flavour and odour that, unlike coconut oil, is also packed with the added health benefits of fibre.*

CREAMY HEMP AND COCONUT PORRIDGE

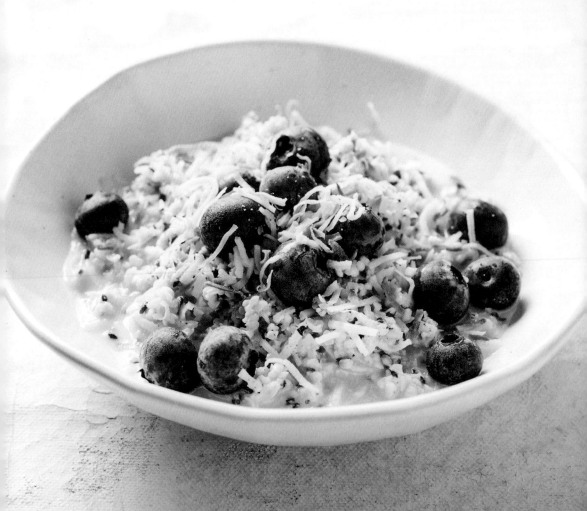

HULLED HEMP SEEDS (ALSO CALLED HEMP HEARTS) ARE A FANTASTIC ALTERNATIVE TO TRADITIONAL OATS, MAKING THIS PORRIDGE RECIPE BOTH GLUTEN FREE AND LOW CARB. YOU DON'T HAVE TO LOOK TOO HARD TO GET YOUR HANDS ON THEM AS THEY CAN BE FOUND IN MOST MAJOR SUPERMARKETS AND HEALTH FOOD STORES.

SERVES 2

250 ml (1 cup) coconut milk
80 g (½ cup) hulled hemp seeds
  (hearts)
3 tablespoons shredded coconut
1 tablespoon coconut oil
½ teaspoon vanilla bean paste
  or powder
¼ teaspoon ground cinnamon
pinch of sea salt
1 tablespoon monk fruit syrup
  or 1–2 drops of liquid stevia
1–2 tablespoons filtered water
  (optional)

TO SERVE
80 g (½ cup) blueberries
1 tablespoon shredded coconut,
  toasted

In a saucepan over medium heat, whisk the coconut milk, hemp seeds, shredded coconut, coconut oil, vanilla, cinnamon, salt and sweetener of choice for 2–3 minutes, or until the mixture begins to bubble. Reduce the heat to low and simmer gently for 10 minutes, or until the mixture is thick and creamy (if it looks too thick, simply add a dash of filtered water).

To serve, divide the porridge between two bowls and top with the blueberries and toasted shredded coconut.

GOOD TO KNOW: *Feel free to mix up the toppings – I also love blackberries, toasted nuts and seeds, and the occasional dollop of nut butter.*

HEALTH HACK: *Hemp hearts are a fantastic plant-based source of protein, omega-3 and omega-6 fatty acids and fibre.*

SEEDED CAULIFLOWER LOAF

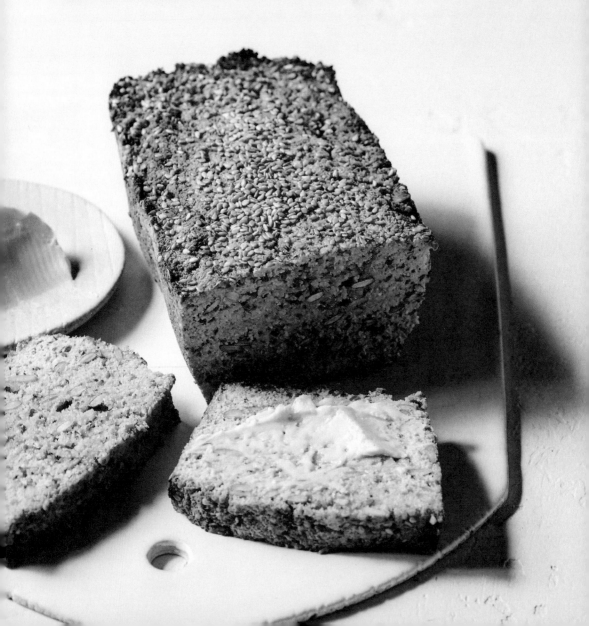

I ABSOLUTELY LOVE THIS RECIPE AS IT'S A GREAT EXAMPLE OF A BREAD THAT IS NUT FREE, LOW CARB AND PACKED WITH THE GOODNESS OF VEGETABLES. WHAT A DELICIOUS MOUTHFUL!

MAKES I LOAF

500 g (about 1 small head) cauliflower, outer leaves removed, broken into small florets
185 ml (¾ cup) coconut oil, melted
6 eggs, at room temperature, plus 1 extra if needed
100 g (¾ cup) coconut flour
1 heaped teaspoon gluten-free baking powder
2 teaspoons sea salt
60 g (½ cup) pumpkin seeds
80 g (½ cup) hulled hemp seeds (hearts)
80 g (½ cup) sesame seeds, plus 1 teaspoon extra
grass-fed butter, to serve (optional)

Preheat the oven to 200°C and line a 22 cm loaf tin with baking paper.

Place the cauliflower florets in a food processor and pulse into tiny rice-like pieces (this usually takes six to eight pulses). Warm 1 tablespoon of the coconut oil in a frying pan over high heat, add the cauliflower rice and saute for 3–4 minutes until softened and light golden brown on the edges. Remove from the heat and set aside.

In a large bowl, whisk the eggs and remaining coconut oil, then add the coconut flour, baking powder and salt and mix well to combine, adding an extra egg if the mixture looks a little dry. Using a spoon, gently stir through the sauteed cauliflower and the seeds.

Spoon the mixture into the prepared loaf tin, sprinkle over the extra sesame seeds and bake for 45 minutes, or until the top is golden brown and the loaf is set. To test, press down gently on the top of the loaf – if it holds its shape, it's ready. Remove from the oven and leave to cool slightly in the tin before turning out, slicing and serving with some butter, if you like.

Store in an airtight container in the fridge for up to 5 days or in the freezer for up to 3 months. If not eating straight away, toast under the grill for best results.

GOOD TO KNOW: *Being completely nut free, this is a fantastic recipe to make for school lunchboxes.*

HEALTH HACK: *I love sneaking pumpkin seeds (AKA pepitas) into as many recipes as I can, as they are a great source of monounsaturated and omega-6 fats.*

BRILLIANT BREAD

THIS IS THE CLOSEST I HAVE EVER COME TO CREATING A RECIPE THAT RESEMBLES 'REAL BREAD'. FIRM AROUND THE EDGES BUT STILL LIGHT AND FLUFFY IN THE MIDDLE, IT'S PERFECT FOR SANDWICHES AND TOASTING.

MAKES 1 LOAF

70 g (½ cup) coconut flour
150 g (1 cup) pumpkin seeds
80 g (1 cup) psyllium husks
3 tablespoons hulled hemp seeds
   (hearts)
3 tablespoons chia seeds
3 tablespoons flax seeds
3 tablespoons sesame seeds
3 teaspoons gluten-free baking
   powder
1 teaspoon sea salt
4 eggs, at room temperature
2 tablespoons coconut oil, melted
1 tablespoon monk fruit syrup, maple
   syrup or coconut nectar
1 tablespoon apple cider vinegar

Preheat the oven to 180°C and line a 22 cm loaf tin with baking paper.

Place the coconut flour, pumpkin seeds, psyllium husks, hemp seeds, chia seeds, flax seeds and sesame seeds in a food processor and blitz to a rough powder. Transfer to a large bowl and stir through the baking powder and salt.

Whisk the eggs in a separate bowl, then whisk in the melted coconut oil, sweetener of choice and apple cider vinegar. Pour the wet ingredients into the dry ingredients and mix well to form a thick, wet dough.

Knead the dough on the bench briefly until springy, then use your hands to roll and shape it into a ball. Gently flatten and stretch the dough lengthways and place it into the prepared loaf tin, using your fingers to push it down into the edges and sides.

Bake for 75–80 minutes or until golden brown and firm to the touch. Remove from the oven and leave to cool slightly, then turn out onto a wire rack and leave to cool completely.

GOOD TO KNOW: *The loaf can be stored in the fridge for up to 7 days or frozen for up to 3 months.*

HEALTH HACK: *It can be tough to find healthy bread at the supermarket, which makes this loaf a game-changer for anyone needing something that is easy, low carb and nut free.*

BANGIN' BUNS

THESE BUNS REALLY ARE BANGIN'! MAKE A BIG BATCH AND HAVE THEM ON HAND FOR WHEN YOU NEED A BREAD ROLL OR A BUN FOR A BURGER LIKE MY 'ZINGER' BURGER ON PAGE 126.

MAKES 8 BUNS

- 100 g (1 cup) almond meal
- 170 g (1¼ cups) coconut flour
- 1 tablespoon psyllium husk powder
- 1 teaspoon sea salt
- 1 teaspoon baking powder
- 2 teaspoons beef gelatine or collagen powder, dissolved in 3 tablespoons boiling water
- 4 egg whites (from large eggs)
- 1 tablespoon apple cider vinegar
- 1 tablespoon monk fruit syrup, maple syrup or raw honey
- 3 tablespoons coconut oil, grass-fed butter or ghee
- 310 ml (1¼ cups) boiling water
- sesame seeds, for sprinkling

Preheat the oven to 180°C and line a baking tray with baking paper.

Place the almond meal, coconut flour, psyllium husk powder, salt and baking powder in a large bowl and mix well.

In a separate bowl, whisk together the dissolved gelatine, egg whites, vinegar and sweetener of choice.

Add the wet ingredients to the dry ingredients, along with the melted coconut oil and boiling water, and mix well to form a dough. Set aside to rest for 2–3 minutes.

Once rested, divide the dough into eight equal portions. Using slightly damp hands, roll one portion into a ball, then transfer it to the prepared baking tray. Repeat with the remaining portions, being sure to space the rolls out evenly on the tray.

Sprinkle the tops of the rolls with the sesame seeds, then bake for 25–30 minutes, or until the rolls are golden brown on top and sound hollow when tapped on the bottom. Remove from the oven, transfer to a wire rack and leave to cool completely before devouring.

GOOD TO KNOW: *These rolls can be stored in the fridge for up to 7 days or frozen for up to 3 months.*

HEALTH HACK: *It can be tough to find healthy rolls at the store, making these rolls perfect for anyone looking for a fuss-free recipe that can be used for lunches, picnics and burgers.*

PUMPKIN AND ZUCCHINI BITES WITH POACHED EGGS AND AVO

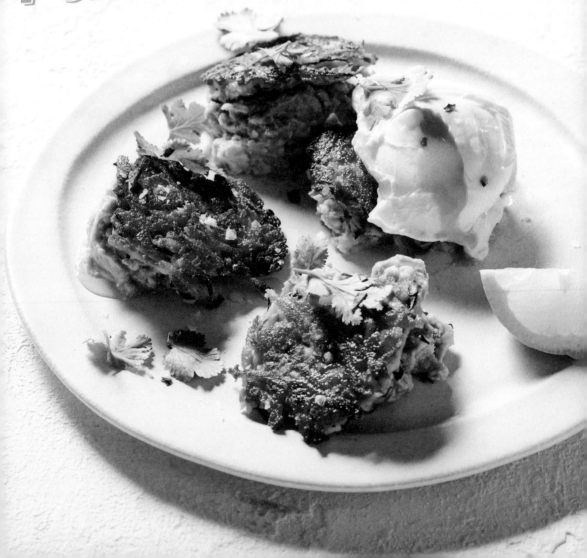

PART FRITTER, PART HASH BROWN, THESE MOUTH-WATERING LITTLE BEAUTIES ARE THE PERFECT SIZE FOR SCOOPING UP ZESTY SMASHED AVO AND DIPPING INTO OOZY EGG YOLKS.

SERVES 4

1 large zucchini
250 g (2 cups) coarsely grated pumpkin
¼ red onion, grated
55 g (½ cup) almond meal, plus extra if needed
1 tablespoon dried chilli flakes
pinch of sea salt
6 eggs
3 tablespoons coconut oil, grass-fed butter or ghee
2 teaspoons apple cider vinegar

SMASHED AVO

2 avocados
finely grated zest and juice of 1 lemon
sea salt

TO SERVE

1 lemon, cut into wedges
1 handful of coriander leaves
sea salt
1 teaspoon dried chilli flakes

For the smashed avo, scoop the avocado flesh into a bowl and gently mash it with the back of a fork. Mix in the lemon zest and juice, season with salt and set aside.

Grate the zucchini and place it on a clean tea towel or muslin cloth, then wrap it up, hold it over the sink and squeeze out the excess liquid until the zucchini is really dry. Alternatively, place the grated zucchini in a colander and squeeze it out over the sink.

Place the zucchini, pumpkin, onion, almond meal, chilli flakes, salt and two of the eggs in a large bowl and mix well to form a batter. If it is looking a little wet, add a touch more almond meal to help it come together.

Melt 1 tablespoon of your preferred cooking fat in a large frying pan over medium heat. Working in batches of five or six at a time, spoon heaped tablespoons of the batter into the pan in loose rounds and press down lightly to form round, bite-sized fritters. Cook for 2–3 minutes on each side until crisp and tender, then transfer to paper towel to drain off any excess oil. Repeat with the remaining fat and batter.

Meanwhile, add the apple cider vinegar to a large saucepan filled with water and bring to the boil. Reduce to a simmer, crack in the remaining four eggs and poach for 4–5 minutes, or until the whites are completely cooked. Carefully remove the eggs from the water with a slotted spoon and transfer to paper towel to remove any excess water.

Divide the pumpkin and zucchini bites, poached eggs and smashed avo among plates and serve with lemon wedges and some coriander leaves. Season with salt and sprinkle over a few extra dried chilli flakes to finish. Enjoy.

GOOD TO KNOW: *Feel free to add some of your favourite herbs or spices to the batter — ground cumin and ground coriander work wonderfully in this recipe.*

HEALTH HACK: *Some people put pumpkin in the same carb bracket as sweet potatoes due to their similarity in look, colour and cooking styles. However, the good news is that pumpkin is a fantastic, naturally sweet low-carb vegetable that can be enjoyed when following a low-carb diet.*

SPICY BREKKIE MUFFINS

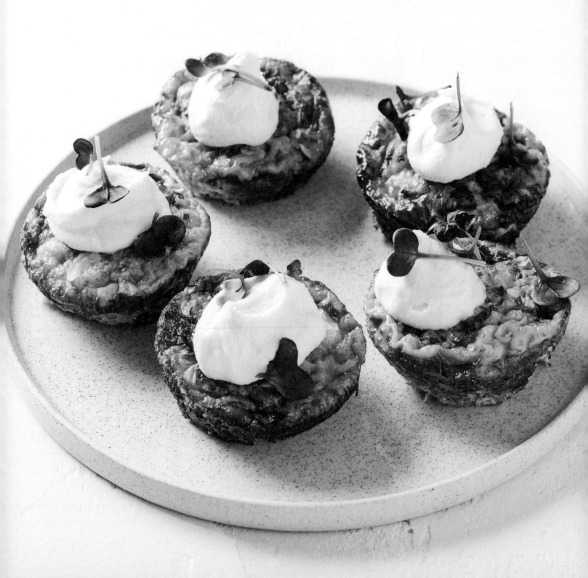

MINI MEAT LOAVES, THAI-STYLE CHICKEN CAKES, HOMEMADE CHOCOLATE … IT'S FAIR TO SAY THERE ISN'T MUCH THAT CAN'T BE MADE IN A HUMBLE MUFFIN TRAY. ALTHOUGH I CALL THESE LITTLE MORSELS MUFFINS, THEY ARE PRETTY MUCH MINI FRITTATAS, AND MAKING THEM IN THE TRAY LIKE THIS MAKES IT AN EASY, NO-STRESS WAY OF WHIPPING UP A BATCH OF MUFFINY GOODNESS. SO WHAT ARE YOU WAITING FOR? IT'S TIME TO GET CRACKING!

MAKES 12

2 tablespoons coconut oil,
    grass-fed butter or ghee, plus
    extra for greasing
2 garlic cloves, finely chopped
½ red onion, finely chopped
1 long red chilli, deseeded and
    finely chopped
1 zucchini, finely diced
¼ head of cauliflower, broken into
    very small florets
8 eggs
50 g (1 cup) baby spinach leaves,
    roughly chopped
sea salt and freshly ground
    black pepper
microherbs, to garnish (optional)

MACADAMIA RICOTTA
(MAKES 500 G OR 1½ CUPS)
320 g (2 cups) macadamia nuts
juice of 1 lemon
1 teaspoon sea salt
125 ml (½ cup) filtered water,
    plus extra if needed

To make the macadamia ricotta, put all the ingredients in a food processor and puree to a smooth paste, scraping down the sides with a spatula halfway through to ensure everything gets mixed well, and adding an extra splash of water if you need to loosen it up a little. Set aside.

Preheat the oven to 180°C and grease a 12-hole muffin tray with your preferred cooking fat.

Heat 2 tablespoons of your preferred cooking fat in a large frying pan over medium heat. Add the garlic, red onion and chilli and saute for 2–3 minutes until softened and lightly caramelised. Add the zucchini and cauliflower and cook, stirring, for another 3–4 minutes until lightly golden. Remove from the heat and set aside.

Whisk the eggs in a bowl until light and fluffy. Add the cooked vegetable mixture and baby spinach, season generously with salt and pepper and mix well to combine.

Spoon the mixture evenly into the prepared muffin tray and bake for 15–20 minutes or until the muffins have risen slightly and a skewer inserted into the centre of each one comes out clean. Leave to cool in the tray for 2 minutes before turning out onto a wire rack to cool completely.

Serve with generous dollops of the macadamia ricotta and some microherbs, if desired.

GOOD TO KNOW: *These muffins can be made in bulk and stored in an airtight container in the fridge for up to 5 days. Leftover ricotta will also keep in an airtight container in the fridge for up to 5 days and is good slathered over a toasted slice of my Seeded Cauliflower Loaf (see page 54).*

HEALTH HACK: *Want to add some animal protein here? Simply throw in a little roughly chopped sausage or bacon when you cook off the vegetable mixture.*

THE BIG BREAKFAST PLATE

SERVES 2

4 portobello mushrooms
1 tablespoon coconut oil, grass-fed
   butter or ghee
4 streaky bacon rashers
4 eggs
200 g (4 cups) baby spinach leaves
1 avocado, quartered
2 tablespoons store-bought
   fermented vegetables (see Good
   to Know)
1 lime, cut into cheeks
sea salt and freshly ground
   black pepper

RED CABBAGE SLAW
¼ red cabbage, finely shredded
1 tablespoon apple cider vinegar
finely grated zest and juice of 1 lime

For the red cabbage slaw, combine all the ingredients in a bowl. Set aside.

Set the oven to grill function with medium heat, position the rack at the top of the oven and line a baking tray with baking paper.

Arrange the mushrooms on the prepared tray bottom-side up and cook for 8–10 minutes, turning halfway through, until charred and softened all over. Set aside.

Meanwhile, melt your preferred cooking fat in a large frying pan over medium–high heat. Add the bacon and cook for 3–4 minutes on each side, or until golden brown and crispy. Remove from the pan and set aside.

Crack the eggs into the same frying pan, reduce the heat to medium and cook for 3–4 minutes until set (doing it this way will use all that delicious bacon fat that remains in the pan). Carefully remove the eggs from the pan and transfer to individual serving plates, sunny-side up.

Add the spinach to the pan and cook, stirring, for 1–2 minutes until gently wilted, then transfer to the serving plates together with the bacon, grilled mushrooms, red cabbage slaw, avocado and fermented veggies. Squeeze over some lime juice, season well with salt and pepper and enjoy.

GOOD TO KNOW: *Feel free to swap out the bacon for a good-quality sausage or even some smoked salmon. When it comes to choosing fermented vegetables, as you can see in this pic I used a turmeric variety that can be found in most health food stores.*

HEALTH HACK: *I have included two delicious versions of cabbage in this recipe in the form of red cabbage slaw and fermented vegetables. Cabbage has an outstanding nutrient profile and is especially high in vitamins C and K. It can also help to improve digestion and combat inflammation.*

I USED TO BE A FAN OF THOSE MASSIVE CAFE-STYLE 'BIG BREAKFASTS' WITH BEEF SAUSAGES, HASH BROWNS AND GIANT PIECES OF THICK-CUT TOAST. HERE'S MY HEALTHY, LOW-CARB ALTERNATIVE FOR THOSE WHO WANT TO BREAK THEIR FAST WITH A BIG FEED WHILE AT THE SAME TIME REAPING THE BENEFITS OF NUTRIENT-DENSE INGREDIENTS.

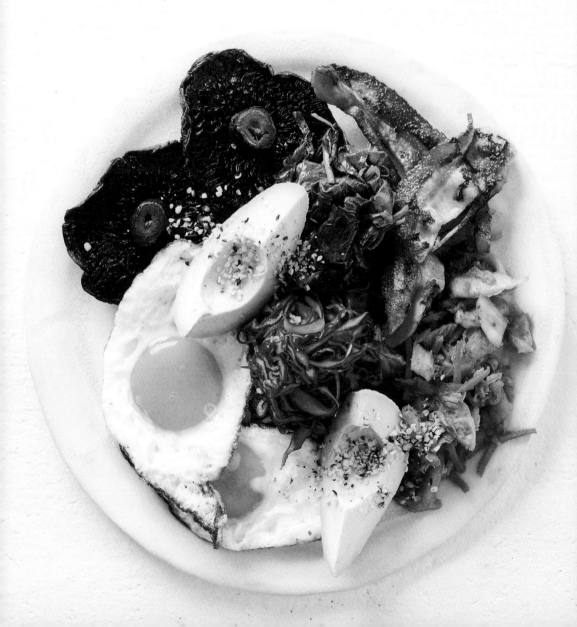

VEGGIE-LOADED MEXICAN FRITTATA

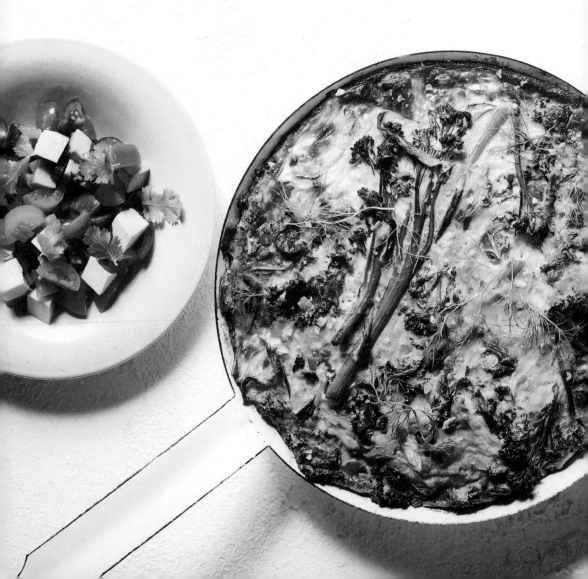

WITH ITS ZESTY FLAVOURS AND SPICY CHILLI KICK, THIS MEXICAN-INSPIRED FRITTATA IS A HARD RECIPE TO GO PAST. WHETHER EATEN FRESH OUT OF THE OVEN OR ENJOYED COLD LATER IN THE WEEK, IT MAKES THE PERFECT BREKKIE … OR ANY OTHER MEAL, FOR THAT MATTER.

SERVES 4–6

2 tablespoons coconut oil, grass-fed
    butter or ghee
2 garlic cloves, finely chopped
2 long red chillies, deseeded
    and finely chopped
½ red onion
2 bunches of broccolini, trimmed
½ fennel bulb, finely sliced
200 g (2 cups) chopped kale
10 eggs
½ teaspoon ground cumin
½ teaspoon ground coriander
sea salt and freshly ground
    black pepper

ZESTY TOMATO AND AVOCADO SALSA

200 g mixed cherry tomatoes,
    quartered
1 avocado, diced
3 tablespoons extra-virgin olive,
    avocado or macadamia oil
1 tablespoon apple cider vinegar
juice of ½ lime
1 small handful of coriander leaves,
    roughly torn

Preheat the oven to 200°C.

Melt your preferred cooking fat in a large ovenproof frying pan over medium–high heat, add the garlic, chilli and red onion and saute for 3–4 minutes until the onion has slightly softened and caramelised. Add the broccolini and fennel and continue to cook, stirring, for 3–4 minutes until softened and lightly browned. Add the kale and saute for 2–3 minutes until it begins to soften. Remove the pan from the heat.

Whisk the eggs together in a bowl along with the cumin, coriander and a pinch of salt and pepper until light and fluffy. Pour the egg mixture into the pan, transfer the pan to the oven and bake for 10–15 minutes, or until the frittata is set. Remove from the oven and leave to cool slightly.

While the frittata is cooling, make the zesty tomato and avocado salsa by combining all the ingredients in a bowl.

Season the frittata generously with salt and pepper and cut it into wedges, then divide among plates and serve with the salsa. Dig in!

GOOD TO KNOW: *If you love chorizo you can easily add it to this recipe – just cut it into small pieces and throw it into the pan when you saute the garlic, onion and chilli. It'll give you some extra protein and healthy fats, bulking things up a little for those looking for a heftier feed.*

HEALTH HACK: *Along with a wide range of beneficial compounds, fennel contains a number of polyphenol antioxidants – potent anti-inflammatory agents that have a positive effect on our health. Reason enough to add a bit more of it to your diet, I reckon!*

JAPANESE OMELETTE

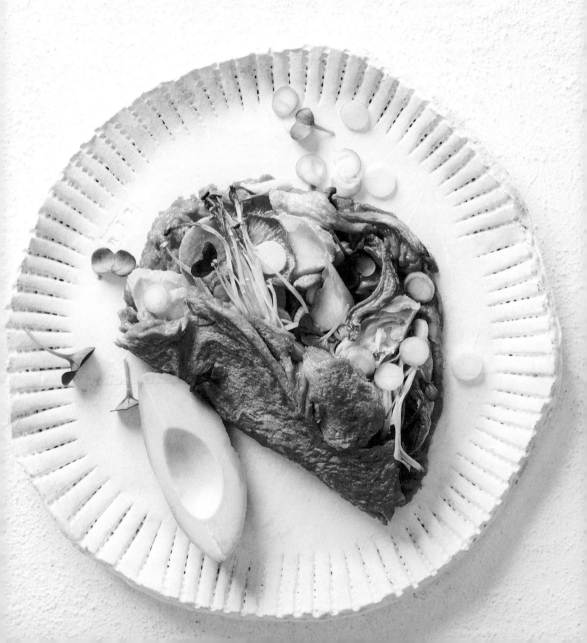

THIS LOVELY OMELETTE HAS A SLIGHTLY DIFFERENT FLAVOUR PROFILE FROM THE ONE YOU MIGHT COOK DAY TO DAY. KEEPING THE MUSHROOMS WHOLE LIKE THIS HELPS GIVE THE FINISHED DISH A CHUNKY, MEATY CONSISTENCY.

SERVES 1

2 tablespoons coconut oil or
grass-fed butter

150 g mixed exotic mushrooms
(shiitake, oyster and enoki
work well)

3 eggs

1 tablespoon coconut aminos
or tamari

50 g hot-smoked salmon fillet,
broken into chunks

1 spring onion, white part only, finely
sliced into rings

1 small handful of Japanese micro
leaves or finely chopped coriander
leaves (optional)

sea salt and freshly ground
black pepper

¼ avocado

Melt 1 tablespoon of your preferred cooking fat in a large frying pan over medium–high heat. Add the mushrooms and saute for 5–6 minutes, stirring and turning often, until softened and lightly golden on all sides. Remove from the pan and set aside.

Whisk the eggs in a bowl with the coconut aminos or tamari until light and fluffy.

Heat the remaining tablespoon of cooking fat in the same pan, then pour in the egg mixture. Using a rubber spatula, gently stir the egg mixture, while tilting the pan and moving it back and forth over the heat. (This keeps the eggs from sticking or browning.) As soon as the egg becomes thick and custardy, stop stirring. Using a spatula, turn the omelette over or, if you're feeling brave, give it a flip! Continue cooking for a further 30 seconds or until cooked through.

To serve, cover one half of the omelette with the cooked mushrooms and salmon pieces, then gently fold it over and top with the spring onion and micro leaves or coriander, if using. Season well with salt and pepper and serve with avocado on the side.

GOOD TO KNOW: *This recipe is really versatile – feel free to swap out the smoked salmon fillet for smoked salmon slices if you prefer, while daikon radish tops, shiso and mizuna leaves all work well as part of the micro leaves here.*

HEALTH HACK: *Mushrooms are great for strengthening the immune system. One of the important ways they do this is by acting as a prebiotic (a food for beneficial bacteria in the gut) helping to support your body's microbiome – the genetic material of all the microbes that live on and inside your body.*

CURRIED SCRAMBLE WITH PUMPKIN WEDGES

SERVES 1

200 g kent pumpkin, deseeded and cut
    into 4 cm thick wedges, skin on
2 tablespoons coconut oil, grass-fed
    butter or ghee
sea salt
1 garlic clove, finely sliced
¼ red onion, finely sliced
1 cm piece of ginger, peeled
    and grated, or ⅛ teaspoon
    ground ginger
1 cm piece of turmeric, grated, or
    ⅛ teaspoon ground turmeric
⅛ teaspoon garam masala
¼ teaspoon dried chilli flakes
3 large eggs
1 small green chilli, deseeded and
    finely sliced
1 small handful of coriander leaves,
    roughly torn

Preheat the oven to 200°C and line a baking tray with baking paper.

Arrange the pumpkin wedges on the prepared tray and coat with 1 tablespoon of your preferred cooking fat. Season well with salt and bake for 15–20 minutes, or until crisp around the edges and cooked through.

Meanwhile, melt the remaining tablespoon of cooking fat in a large frying pan over medium heat. Add the garlic and onion and saute for 2–3 minutes until softened and caramelised, then add the ginger, turmeric, garam masala and chilli flakes. Season well with salt and cook for a further 2–3 minutes, stirring, until aromatic.

Whisk the eggs in a large bowl until light and fluffy.

Reduce the heat to medium–low and pour the beaten egg into the pan. Gently keep the eggs moving, stirring and scraping the sides of the pan until the scramble is creamy and holding its form, about 2–3 minutes. Remove from the heat (the eggs will continue to cook once off the heat, so be careful not to overcook them here).

Place the pumpkin wedges on a plate, spoon over the scramble, scatter over the green chilli and coriander and serve immediately.

GOOD TO KNOW: *The kent variety of pumpkin (also known as kabocha) is easily identified by its green skin, mottled with yellow and brown patches, and bright orange flesh.*

HEALTH HACK: *Spices really are your best friends in the kitchen – they help make food taste incredible and add many health boosting properties to your plate. Chillies, for example, can help fight inflammation, clear congestion and boost immunity.*

THIS RECIPE IS BASED ON A TRADITIONAL NORTH INDIAN BREAKFAST THAT PAIRS AROMATIC SCRAMBLED EGGS WITH FRESHLY MADE FLATBREADS. HERE I'VE SWAPPED OUT THE FLATBREADS FOR OVEN-ROASTED PUMPKIN WEDGES, WHICH I THINK GO REALLY WELL WITH THE FLAVOURS OF THIS DISH.

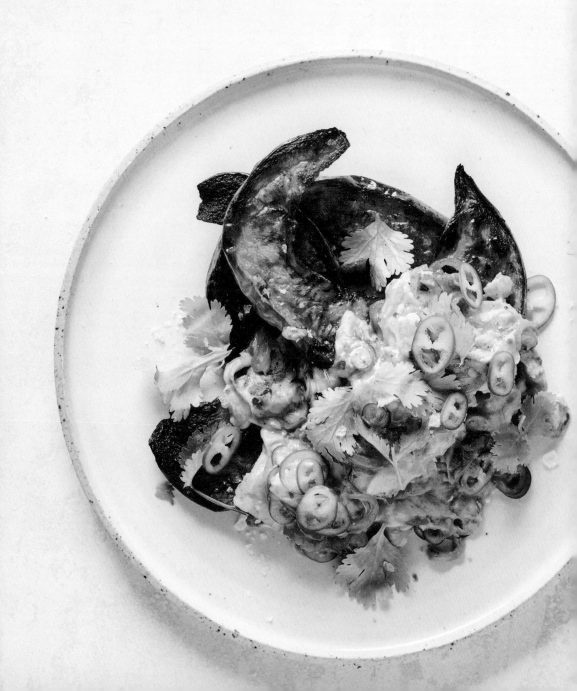

VEGET

ABLES

LOADED AVOCADOS WITH LEMONY DREAM CHEESE

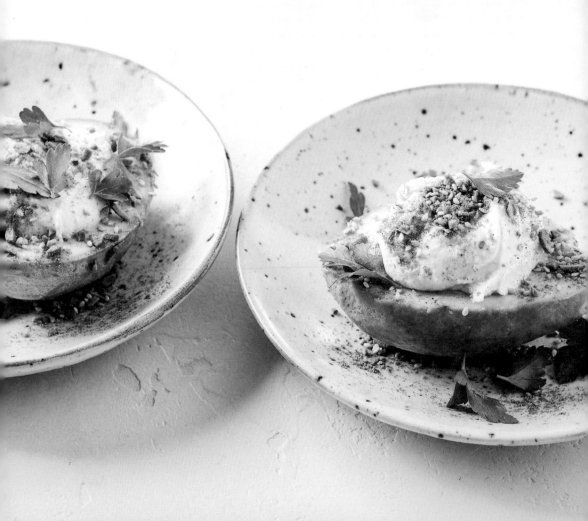

I AM ALWAYS LOOKING FOR NEW WAYS TO INCORPORATE AVOCADO INTO MY DIET. THIS ONE TICKS ALL THE RIGHT DELICIOUS BOXES AND, IF YOU MAKE UP THE DUKKAH AND DREAM CHEESE IN ADVANCE, YOU CAN THROW IT TOGETHER IN NO TIME AT ALL. YOU'LL HAVE LEFTOVER DUKKAH AFTER MAKING THIS RECIPE BUT THAT'S NO BIGGIE — IT'S ALSO GREAT WITH THE CHARGRILLED ZUCCHINI ON PAGE 82 AND THE CAULIFLOWER/BROCCOLI STEAKS ON PAGE 84.

SERVES 4

2 avocados, halved
80 ml (⅓ cup) extra-virgin olive oil
2 tablespoons flat-leaf parsley leaves
sea salt and freshly ground
    black pepper

DUKKAH

3 tablespoons sesame seeds
70 g (½ cup) pistachio kernels,
    finely chopped
3 teaspoons ground coriander
3 teaspoons ground cumin
½ teaspoon freshly ground
    black pepper
1 teaspoon sea salt

LEMONY DREAM CHEESE

240 g (1½ cups) macadamia nuts or
    cashew nuts
3 tablespoons canned coconut milk
    or coconut cream
2 tablespoons apple cider vinegar
finely grated zest and juice of 1 lemon
½ teaspoon sea salt

Get started on the dukkah. Toast the sesame seeds in a non-stick frying pan over medium heat for 5 minutes, or until golden. Add the pistachios, ground spices and pepper and cook, stirring, for 1 minute until aromatic. Stir in the salt and set aside to cool.

For the dream cheese, place all the ingredients in a food processor or high-speed blender and blitz until smooth and creamy.

To serve, arrange the avocado halves cut-side up on individual serving plates and fill the holes of each with a tablespoon or so of dream cheese. Drizzle over the olive oil, sprinkle over the dukkah and parsley and season with salt and pepper. Tuck in.

GOOD TO KNOW: *To give the dream cheese a really smooth finish, try soaking the nuts in hot water for 1 hour, then drain before blending. Any leftover dream cheese is excellent slathered over toasted slices of my Seeded Cauliflower Loaf (see page 54).*

HEALTH HACK: *This recipe combines some of my favourite healthy fats in the form of avocados, extra-virgin olive oil and omega-3 rich nuts. This combination of nutrient-dense ingredients will reduce cravings and make you feel satiated.*

RAW RAINBOW RIBBONS

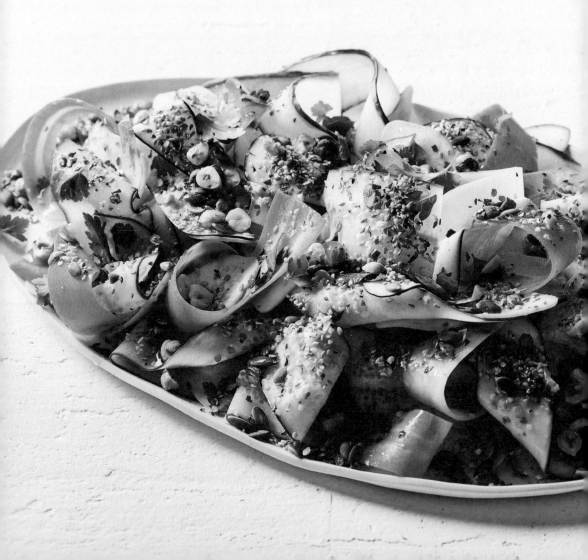

I LOVE THE CRISP CRUNCH THAT RAW VEGETABLES HAVE — COMBINE THEM WITH AN EASY DRESSING AND SOME TEXTURE FROM NUTS AND SEEDS AND YOU'RE ONTO A WINNER. THIS DISH IS SIMPLE AND COLOURFUL, PLUS IT CAN BE WHIPPED UP IN MOMENTS. I RECOMMEND YOU INVEST IN A GOOD-QUALITY MANDOLINE OR PEELER THAT WILL GIVE YOU CONSISTENT RIBBONS WITH YOUR VEGETABLES, BUT FAILING THAT A VERY SHARP KNIFE WILL DO.

SERVES 4

1 continental cucumber
1 carrot
2 zucchini (a mix of colours is lovely)
½ green papaya (paw paw), peeled
1 bunch of flat-leaf parsley, leaves
    roughly torn

DRESSING
125 ml (½ cup) extra-virgin olive,
    avocado or macadamia oil
finely grated zest and juice of
    2 lemons
2 tablespoons apple cider vinegar
1 tablespoon dried chilli flakes
½ teaspoon sea salt

TOASTED NUT AND SEED TOPPING
70 g (½ cup) hazelnuts,
    roughly chopped
2 tablespoons sesame seeds
2 tablespoons hulled hemp seeds
    (hearts)
2 tablespoons pumpkin seeds

To make the dressing, place all the ingredients in a bowl or jar and whisk or shake well to combine.

For the toasted nut and seed topping, place the ingredients in a dry frying pan over medium heat and toast for 3–4 minutes, tossing the pan regularly, until lightly golden brown and aromatic. Set aside to cool.

Using a mandoline, vegetable peeler or very sharp knife, cut the vegetables and papaya into thin ribbons. Transfer the ribbons and parsley to a large bowl, pour over the dressing and toss well to combine.

To serve, pile the dressed rainbow ribbons onto a large platter and sprinkle over the toasted nut and seed topping to finish.

GOOD TO KNOW: *You might be wondering what the difference is between a regular papaya, or paw paw, and a green one. Well a green papaya is simply a papaya that is picked while unripe. It is awesome shredded or cut into ribbons in salads like this, or even added to curries.*

HEALTH HACK: *I love including apple cider vinegar as a form of acid in my salad dressings, not only because of the wonderful zing it adds to a dish but also because the main substance in the vinegar, acetic acid, can help kill harmful bacteria or prevent them from multiplying.*

BABY SPINACH SALAD WITH MINTY CASHEW DRESSING

SERVES 4

4 large handfuls of baby spinach leaves
1 handful of mint leaves
1 handful of flat-leaf parsley leaves,
    roughly torn
½ red onion, finely sliced
sea salt and freshly ground
    black pepper

DRESSING

3 tablespoons roughly chopped
    mint leaves
3 tablespoons finely chopped
    cashew nuts
125 ml (½ cup) extra-virgin olive or
    avocado oil
finely grated zest and juice of 1 lemon
1 tablespoon apple cider vinegar
1 tablespoon dijon mustard

For the dressing, place all the ingredients in a bowl and whisk to combine.

In a separate large bowl, toss together the baby spinach leaves, mint, parsley and red onion. Season well with salt and pepper, pour over the dressing and toss to coat. Serve.

GOOD TO KNOW: *This recipe lends itself well to being made in bulk and can be prepared in advance — simply store the salad ingredients separately from the dressing, then toss them together shortly before serving.*

HEALTH HACK: *Spinach really is a superfood. As well as providing a great source of protein and iron, these dark leafy greens are loaded with tons of vitamins, minerals and other nutrients that are important for skin, hair and bone health.*

IT WOULD BE REMISS OF ME NOT TO INCLUDE A RECIPE THAT CHAMPIONS ONE OF THE MOST COMMONLY PURCHASED SALAD LEAVES OUT THERE, THE HUMBLE BABY SPINACH LEAF. THIS RELATIVELY CHEAP STAPLE IS PACKED FULL OF WONDERFUL NUTRIENTS AND HAS A DELICIOUS MILD FLAVOUR THAT MAKES IT PERFECT FOR THE WHOLE FAMILY — JUST WAIT TILL YOU TRY IT WITH THIS MINTY CASHEW DRESSING!

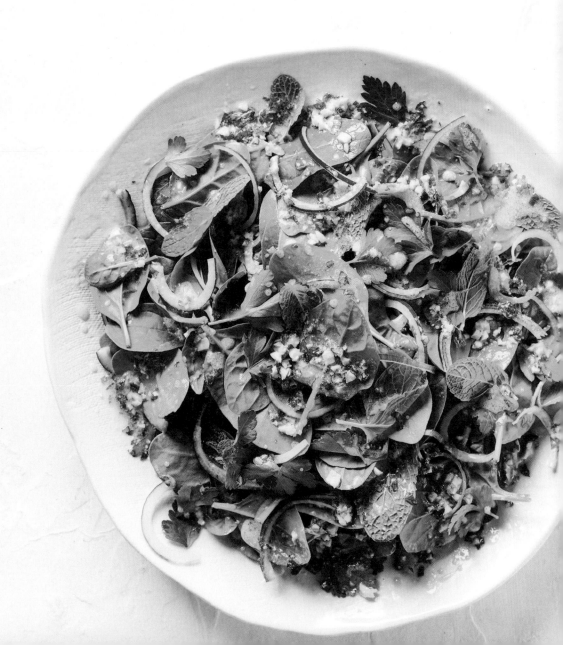

GORGEOUS GREEN TABBOULEH

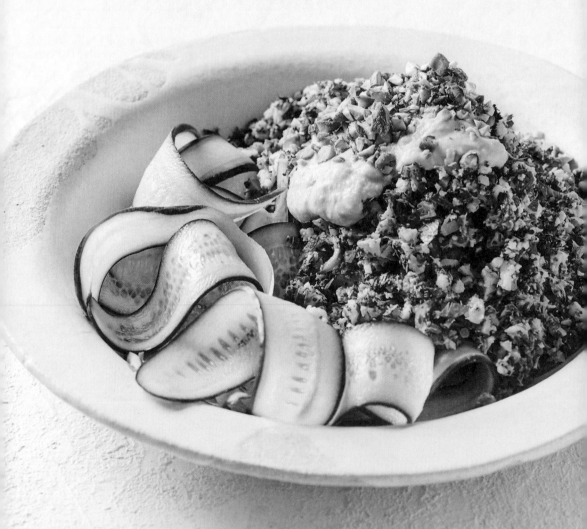

TABBOULEH IS A SIMPLE MEDITERRANEAN SALAD OF VERY FINELY CHOPPED VEGETABLES, LOTS OF FRESH PARSLEY AND BULGUR WHEAT, ALL TOSSED TOGETHER WITH LEMON JUICE AND OLIVE OIL. MY TAKE CELEBRATES ALL THE GOODNESS OF THE PARSLEY, LEMON JUICE AND OLIVE OIL, BUT SWITCHES OUT THE BULGUR WHEAT FOR TWO GRAIN-FREE, LOW-CARB ALTERNATIVES — BROCCOLI AND CAULIFLOWER RICE.

SERVES 4

3 heads of broccoli (about 800 g
   in total), broken into florets and
   roughly chopped
¼ head of cauliflower, broken into
   florets and roughly chopped
2 garlic cloves, chopped
1 tablespoon extra-virgin olive oil
sea salt and freshly ground
   black pepper
2 handfuls of flat-leaf parsley leaves,
   finely chopped
1 handful of mint leaves,
   finely chopped,
1 long green chilli, finely sliced
1 Lebanese cucumber
3 tablespoons pistachio kernels,
   toasted and roughly chopped

DRESSING
1 avocado
3 tablespoons extra-virgin olive oil
3 tablespoons coconut yoghurt
finely grated zest and juice of 1 lemon
sea salt and freshly ground
   black pepper

Preheat the oven to 220°C and line two baking trays with baking paper.

Working in batches if necessary, place the broccoli and cauliflower in a food processor and pulse into tiny rice-like pieces (this usually takes six to eight pulses). Transfer to a large bowl, add the garlic and oil, season with salt and pepper and stir to combine. Spread the mixture over the prepared baking trays in an even layer and bake for 8–10 minutes, or until lightly golden brown. Remove from the oven and set aside to cool.

Meanwhile, make the dressing. Halve the avocado, scoop out the flesh and add it to a food processor together with the oil, yoghurt, lemon zest and juice. Blitz everything together until smooth and creamy, then season with salt and pepper and set aside.

Once cool, transfer the cooked cauliflower and broccoli to a large bowl and add the parsley, mint and chilli. Pour over half of the dressing and toss to combine.

Using a mandoline, vegetable peeler or very sharp knife, cut the cucumber into thin ribbons, then divide it among serving plates. Add the tabbouleh, then spoon over the remaining dressing and sprinkle over the toasted pistachios. Season with salt and pepper and enjoy.

GOOD TO KNOW: *This recipe calls for pistachio kernels. These are raw, shelled and unsalted pistachios. You can find these in most supermarkets and health food stores.*

HEALTH HACK: *I love to use pistachios in my cooking as they are high in fibre, which is good for your gut bacteria, plus they are among the most antioxidant-rich nuts around.*

MAGNIFICENT MUSHROOM SKEWERS

SERVES 2

3 tablespoons extra-virgin olive oil
1 teaspoon dried chilli flakes
½ teaspoon smoked paprika
1 teaspoon finely chopped fresh or
    dried rosemary
finely grated zest and juice of 1 lemon
16 brown mushrooms
sea salt and freshly ground
    black pepper
1 red onion, quartered

CHIMICHURRI

1 bunch of coriander, leaves
    roughly torn
1 bunch of flat-leaf parsley, leaves
    roughly torn
2 garlic cloves, roughly chopped
¼ red onion, roughly chopped
1 long red chilli, deseeded and
    roughly chopped
1 teaspoon dried oregano
3 tablespoons extra-virgin olive oil
1 tablespoon apple cider vinegar

GARLIC FLATBREADS

55 g (½ cup) almond meal
60 g (½ cup) arrowroot or
    tapioca flour
¼ teaspoon garlic powder
3 tablespoons coconut milk
3 tablespoons filtered water
pinch of sea salt
2–3 tablespoons coconut oil

Place four bamboo skewers in a shallow dish, cover with cold water and leave to soak for at least 30 minutes.

To make the chimichurri, blitz all the ingredients in a food processor until smooth. Spoon into a bowl and set aside in the fridge until ready to serve.

In a large bowl, whisk together the olive oil, chilli flakes, paprika, rosemary, lemon zest and juice. Add the mushrooms to the bowl and toss to coat, then season with a little salt and pepper. Set aside while you make your flatbreads.

For the flatbreads, combine the almond meal, arrowroot or tapioca flour, garlic powder, coconut milk, water and salt in a bowl and mix well to form a smooth, thinnish batter. (The more watery the batter, the thinner and crispier your flatbreads will be, so add a splash or two more if you like.)

Melt 1 tablespoon of the coconut oil in a small non-stick frying pan over medium heat. Ladle one-quarter of the batter into the pan, tilting and swirling it to coat the base in an even layer, and cook for 2–3 minutes, then carefully turn the flatbread over with a spatula and cook for a further 2 minutes, or until golden and cooked through. Lift the flatbread from the pan and wrap in a clean tea towel to keep warm. Repeat with the remaining batter, greasing the pan with coconut oil in between to make sure the flatbreads don't stick to the pan. Set aside in a low oven to keep warm.

Preheat a barbecue or chargrill pan to high.

Thread the mushrooms and red onion evenly onto the skewers and grill for 10–15 minutes, turning every 2–3 minutes, until charred on all sides and cooked through. Serve with the flatbreads and chimichurri.

GOOD TO KNOW: *Any leftover chimichurri will keep in an airtight container in the fridge for up to 7 days. It is also incredible spooned over roast vegetables or with steak (see page 148).*

YOU'LL BE A MUSHROOM MASTER ONCE YOU NAIL THIS QUICK AND EASY RECIPE.
I LIKE TO KEEP THESE SKEWERS ALL ABOUT THE MUSHROOMS BUT FEEL FREE TO
ADD SOME OF YOUR OTHER FAVOURITE ABOVE-GROUND VEGETABLES, SUCH AS
ZUCCHINI OR EGGPLANT.

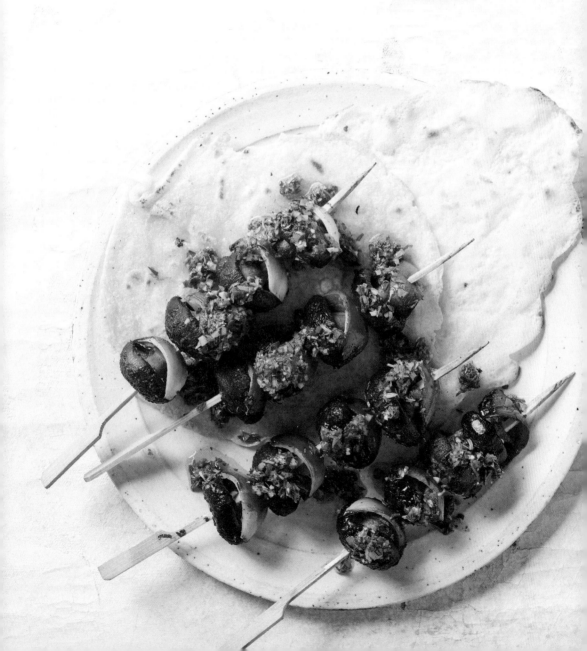

CHARGRILLED ZUCCHINI with AVOCADO HUMMUS

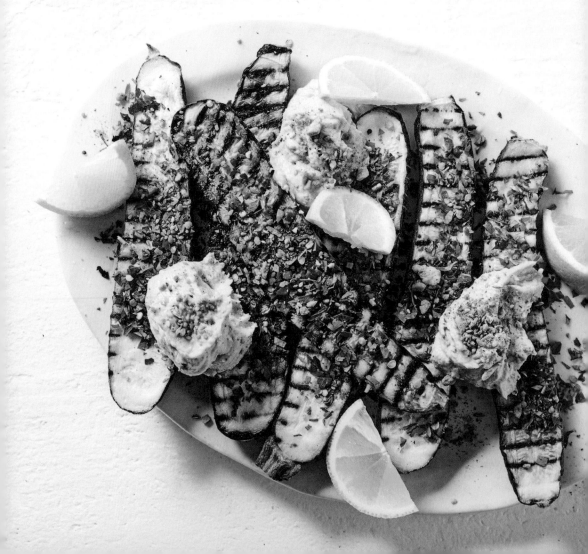

THIS RECIPE IS DELICIOUSLY FRESH AND LIGHT — I JUST LOVE THE CONTRASTING TEXTURES AND FLAVOURS OF THE CHARRED ZUCCHINI, CREAMY AVOCADO HUMMUS AND CRUNCHY DUKKAH. I LIKE TO USE A MIX OF YELLOW AND GREEN ZUCCHINI HERE FOR COLOUR, BUT FEEL FREE TO USE WHATEVER YOU LIKE!

SERVES 4

6 small zucchini (about 1 kg in total),
   halved lengthways
1 garlic clove, crushed
finely grated zest and juice of 1 lemon
3 tablespoons extra-virgin olive oil,
   plus extra to serve
pinch each of sea salt and freshly
   ground black pepper
½ bunch of flat-leaf parsley, leaves
   finely chopped
½ teaspoon dried chilli flakes
3 tablespoons Dukkah (see page 73)
lemon wedges, to serve

AVOCADO HUMMUS

2 avocados
135 g (½ cup) hulled tahini
1 garlic clove, crushed
finely grated zest and juice of 1 lemon
3 tablespoons extra-virgin olive oil
sea salt and freshly ground
   black pepper

To make the avocado hummus, blitz the avocado, tahini, garlic, lemon zest and juice and olive oil in a food processor until smooth and creamy. Season to taste with salt and pepper and set aside.

Heat a large chargrill pan or barbecue grill to high. Cook the zucchini halves, in batches if necessary, for 3 minutes on each side, or until charred and cooked through.

While the zucchini is cooking, mix the garlic, lemon zest and juice, oil, salt and pepper in a large bowl.

When all the zucchini slices are cooked, gently toss them in the garlic dressing, then pile them onto a serving platter. Scatter over the parsley and chilli flakes, finish with generous dollops of the avocado hummus and sprinkle over the dukkah. Serve with lemon wedges for squeezing.

GOOD TO KNOW: *Dukkah is a great addition to salads and roast vegetables, so feel free to make a big batch and store it in an airtight container in the pantry for up to 3 months.*

HEALTH HACK: *Move over chia seeds and spirulina, the humble avocado has got to be one of the original and best superfoods out there. Containing a wide variety of nutrients, including 20 different vitamins and minerals, it is also packed with fibre and is one of my favourite sources of healthy fat.*

SENSATIONAL SUMAC STEAKS

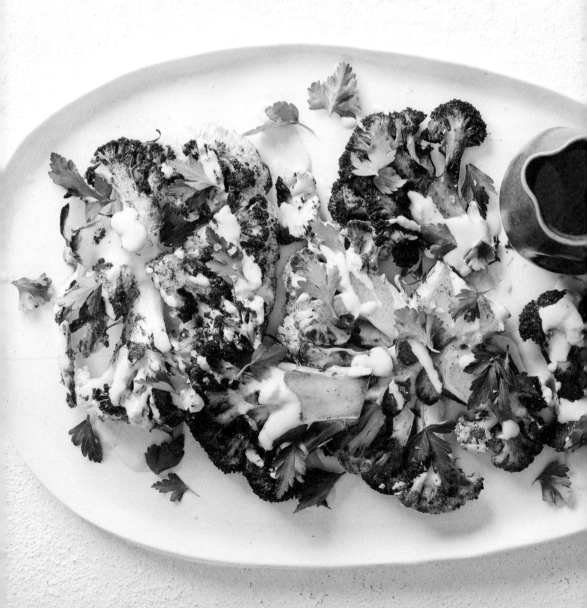

BECAUSE WE EAT WITH OUR EYES, I ALWAYS AIM TO MAKE MY RECIPES LOOK AS IRRESISTIBLE AS POSSIBLE, AND THESE SUMAC STEAKS REALLY ARE A PRETTY PICTURE. TRY WHIPPING THEM UP YOURSELF AND YOUR MEAT-FREE MONDAYS WILL SOON BE LOOKING BETTER THAN EVER!

SERVES 4

1 head of cauliflower
1 large head of broccoli
2 tablespoons coconut oil
125 ml (½ cup) extra-virgin olive oil
1 tablespoon sumac
1 teaspoon ground cumin
½ teaspoon chilli powder
½ teaspoon garlic powder
sea salt and freshly ground
    black pepper
1 handful of flat-leaf parsley leaves,
    roughly chopped

DRESSING

2 tablespoons hulled tahini
125 g (½ cup) coconut yoghurt or
    canned coconut cream
125 ml (½ cup) lemon juice
sea salt and freshly ground
    black pepper

Preheat the oven to 180°C and line two baking trays with baking paper.

Sit the cauliflower upright on a chopping board and cut four even slices about 4 cm thick out of the centre. Repeat with the broccoli.

Melt the coconut oil in a large frying pan over high heat. Add a few of the cauliflower and broccoli steaks to the pan and fry for 6–8 minutes, turning halfway through, or until nicely caramelised. Transfer the steaks to one of the prepared trays and repeat with the remaining cauliflower and broccoli.

In a small bowl, whisk the olive oil, sumac, cumin, chilli and garlic powder. Drizzle this mixture over the cauliflower and broccoli steaks to coat evenly and season well with salt and pepper. Roast for 20–30 minutes, or until the steaks are soft on the inside and golden brown on the edges.

Meanwhile, for the dressing, whisk all the ingredients in a bowl. Set aside.

To serve, divide the cauliflower and broccoli steaks among plates, giving each person one of each. Top with a generous drizzle of the dressing and a scattering of chopped parsley.

GOOD TO KNOW: *This is a fantastic recipe to use any leftover dukkah from the Loaded Avocados on page 72. Sprinkle a little over the top before serving.*

HEALTH HACK: *Tahini is a condiment made from toasted ground sesame seeds. Used in the cuisines of the Middle East and parts of North Africa, it contains more protein than milk and most nuts, is a rich source of the B vitamins that boost energy and brain function, and is packed with important minerals, such as magnesium, iron and calcium.*

BAKED BUTTERNUT FRIES

SERVES 4

1 butternut pumpkin
2 tablespoons extra-virgin olive oil
1 tablespoon dried rosemary
1 tablespoon sweet paprika
1 tablespoon arrowroot or
  tapioca flour
sea salt and freshly ground
  black pepper

SPICY MAYO

3 tablespoons No-fail Plant-based
  Mayo (see page 127)
½ teaspoon chilli powder, or to taste

Preheat the oven to 200°C and line a large baking tray with baking paper.

Halve the pumpkin vertically and scoop out the seeds, then remove the skin with a vegetable peeler or sharp knife, reserving it if you like (see Good to Know). Cut the pumpkin halves horizontally into 1.5 cm thick half-moons, then cut each half-moon into 5 mm thick pieces.

Add the butternut pieces to a bowl together with the oil, rosemary, paprika and arrowroot or tapioca flour and toss to coat evenly. Season well with salt and pepper.

Spread the coated butternut pieces evenly across the prepared tray, making sure they don't overlap (use a second tray if you need to here — it's important that the fries cook in a single layer). Bake for 25–35 minutes, turning halfway through, until golden brown and crispy on the outside and soft in the middle.

To make the spicy mayo, mix the ingredients in a small bowl.

Remove the fries from the oven and season generously with sea salt. Serve with the spicy mayo for dipping.

GOOD TO KNOW: *I like to reserve the pumpkin skin and bake it separately with a good-quality cooking fat until charred — these make great crisps! Be careful, though, as they cook quickly and can burn more easily than the fries.*

HEALTH HACK: *Bananas are always celebrated for their high levels of potassium, but did you know that a cup of cubed butternut pumpkin provides 582 mg of potassium, which is more than the amount found in a banana? Just one of the many reasons this delicious low-carb veg is one of my all-time faves!*

I LOVE FRIES BUT, WHEN GOING LOW CARB, I TRY TO REDUCE MY INTAKE OF THE STARCHY BELOW-GROUND ROOT VEGETABLES THAT ARE MOST COMMONLY USED TO MAKE THEM. SO HERE I'M INTRODUCING … BAKED BUTTERNUT FRIES! AS WELL AS BEING DELICIOUS, THESE ARE PACKED WITH AN ABUNDANCE OF NUTRITION AND ARE REALLY SIMPLE TO MAKE. BELIEVE ME, YOU'VE JUST GOTTA TRY THESE.

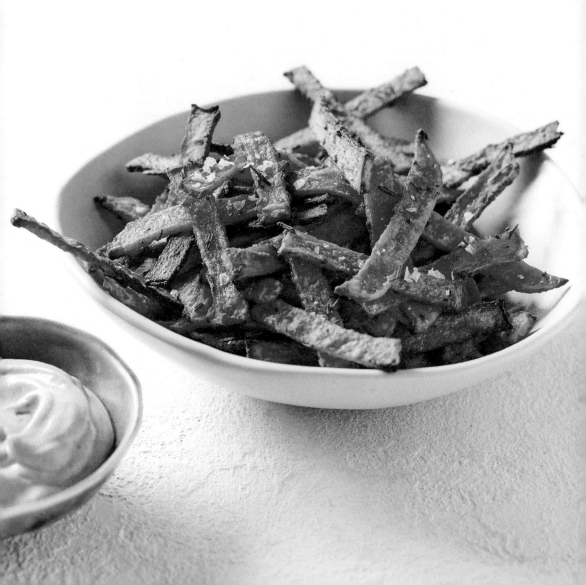

SPICY BROCCOLI PAKORA

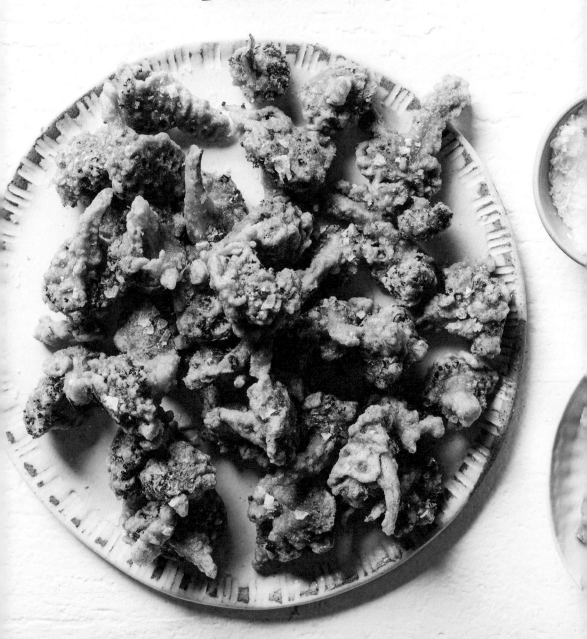

IF YOU LOVE BROCCOLI, THEN THIS VERSION OF THE CLASSIC NORTH INDIAN VEGETARIAN SNACK IS AN ABSOLUTE MUST! THESE CRISPY, BITE-SIZED MORSELS ARE SUCH AN EASY YET INDULGENT WAY TO ENJOY THIS SUPER VEG. THEY MAKE THE PERFECT SNACK AS THEY ARE BUT ARE ALSO GREAT MADE UP IN A LARGE BATCH AND SERVED ON A PLATTER WITH SOME SPICY MAYO (SEE PAGE 86) FOR A DINNER PARTY.

SERVES 4

1 head of broccoli, cut into
    very small florets
125 ml (½ cup) coconut oil
sea salt

SPICY BATTER

3 tablespoons coconut flour,
    plus extra if necessary
2 tablespoons arrowroot
    or tapioca flour
1 teaspoon chilli powder
1 teaspoon ground coriander
1 teaspoon ground cumin
1 teaspoon ground turmeric
generous pinch of sea salt
250 ml (1 cup) filtered water

To make the batter, place the flours, spices and salt in a large bowl and mix well. Pour over the water, whisking all the while to avoid lumps, to form a smooth, thick batter. (If the batter is looking too thin, add a little extra coconut flour.)

Add the broccoli florets to the batter and coat well using your hands.

Melt the coconut oil in a deep frying pan over medium–high heat until nice and hot. To see if the oil is hot enough, add a small battered floret as a test – if it sizzles straight away, you're good to go!

Fry the battered florets in small batches for 4–5 minutes, until nicely browned, lowering them into the hot oil one at a time, spacing them out and being careful not to overcrowd the pan. Remove the cooked pakora with a slotted spoon and set aside on paper towel to drain, then repeat with the remaining florets. (Don't freak out if some of the batter sticks to the pan or comes off – this is normal.)

Serve warm with a generous pinch or two of salt.

GOOD TO KNOW: *This recipe also works really well with cauliflower, so feel free to sub out the broccoli or simply do a delicious combination of both.*

HEALTH HACK: *Broccoli is a nutrient-rich vegetable that can enhance your health in a variety of ways, such as reducing inflammation, improving blood sugar control, boosting immunity and promoting heart health.*

MINI VEGGIE PIES

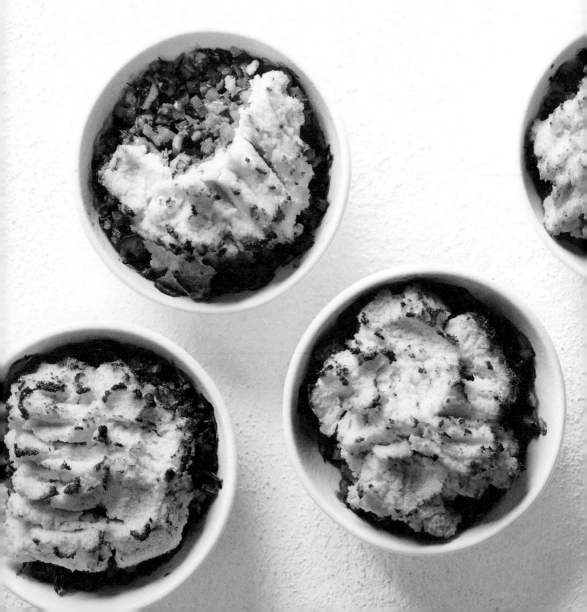

THESE LITTLE INDIVIDUAL PIES PRESENT BEAUTIFULLY BUT YOU CAN ALWAYS ASSEMBLE THIS IN ONE LARGE CASSEROLE DISH AND SERVE IT IN THE MIDDLE OF THE TABLE IF YOU PREFER.

SERVES 4

1 small head of cauliflower (about 600 g), broken into small florets
1 head of broccoli (about 200 g), broken into small florets and roughly chopped
80 ml (⅓ cup) extra-virgin olive or avocado oil, plus extra for drizzling
1 onion, finely diced
2 carrots, finely diced
1 celery stalk, finely diced
4 garlic cloves, very finely chopped
500 g Swiss brown mushrooms, roughly chopped
1 tablespoon tomato paste
250 ml (1 cup) vegetable stock or chicken or beef bone broth (see Health Hack)
3 tablespoons nutritional yeast
1 tablespoon dijon mustard
1 tablespoon roughly chopped thyme leaves
sea salt and freshly ground black pepper

Preheat the oven to 200°C.

Bring a large saucepan of salted water to the boil, add the cauliflower and boil for 5–6 minutes or until lovely and tender. Drain and set aside.

Place the broccoli in a food processor and pulse into tiny rice-like pieces (this usually takes six to eight pulses). Set aside.

Warm 2 tablespoons of your chosen oil in a large frying pan over medium heat, add the onion, carrot, celery and garlic and cook, stirring, for 4–5 minutes or until golden and caramelised. Add the broccoli 'rice' and saute for a further 4–5 minutes, until softened, then add the mushroom in batches, making sure not to add it all at once and giving each batch a chance to soften down a little before adding the next. Stir in the tomato paste and cook for a further 2 minutes, then increase the heat to high, add the vegetable stock or bone broth and bring to the boil. Reduce the heat to low and simmer for 5–10 minutes, or until the liquid has reduced by roughly half. Remove from the heat.

Place the cauliflower in a food processor or high-powered blender along with the remaining 2 tablespoons of oil and the nutritional yeast, mustard and thyme leaves. Blend to a smooth mash, then season to taste with salt and pepper.

Divide the vegetable mixture among four large ramekins and top each with the cauliflower mash. Drizzle a little oil over the top and bake for 20 minutes or until lightly golden. Serve.

GOOD TO KNOW: *I have used cauliflower to top this pie, but feel free to use pumpkin instead. The recipe stays the same — just boil your chosen vegetable for long enough that it will blend well in the food processor.*

HEALTH HACK: *If you're vegetarian or vegan you should simply use a vegetable stock here. But if you're not, I love the flavour that a good chicken or beef bone broth brings to this dish — plus all the nutritional benefits of collagen and gelatine for gut health and improved skin, hair and nails, of course.*

ZESTY ZUCCHINI WITH PINE NUT AND PUMPKIN SEED CRUMB

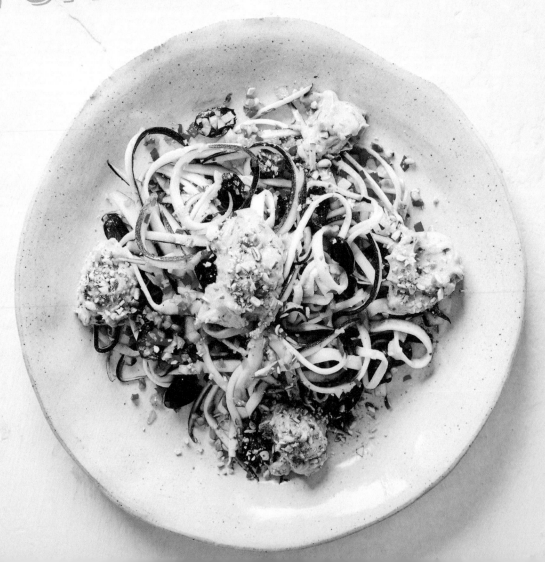

THIS MAKES A FANTASTIC HEALTHY LUNCH ON ITS OWN, BUT IS ALSO A GREAT SIDE DISH TO ACCOMPANY YOUR FAVOURITE PROTEIN, SUCH AS THE RAS-EL-HANOUT CHICKEN ON PAGE 122 OR THE SALMON FISHCAKES ON PAGE 98.

SERVES 4

3 tablespoons pine nuts
3 tablespoons pumpkin seeds
2 zucchini
2 tablespoons coconut oil
½ onion, finely chopped
2 garlic cloves, finely chopped
1 long red chilli, deseeded and
    finely chopped
12 kalamata olives, pitted and halved
sea salt and freshly ground
    black pepper
zest and juice of 1 lemon

AVOCADO DRESSING
125 ml (½ cup) extra-virgin olive,
    avocado, macadamia or hemp oil
1 avocado
1 handful of coriander leaves
1 tablespoon apple cider vinegar
1 teaspoon chilli powder
finely grated zest and juice of 1 lime
pinch of sea salt

Preheat the oven to 180°C and line a large baking tray with baking paper.

Spread the pine nuts and pumpkin seeds evenly across the prepared tray and roast for 8–10 minutes, turning halfway through cooking, or until aromatic and lightly golden. Remove from the oven and leave to cool slightly, then roughly chop until the mixture resembles a crumb. Set aside.

For the avocado dressing, blitz all the ingredients in a food processor until smooth and creamy. Set aside.

Using a mandoline or sharp knife, cut the zucchini into thin strips, then cut each strip lengthways into noodles. Alternatively, you can use a spiraliser to create your zucchini noodles.

Melt the coconut oil in a large frying pan over medium heat. Add the onion, garlic and chilli and saute for 2 minutes, or until the onion is translucent and everything is nicely aromatic. Add the olives and cook, stirring gently, for a further 2 minutes, then add the zucchini noodles and stir gently to coat them in all the lovely flavours. Season to taste with salt and pepper.

Divide the warm zucchini noodles among serving bowls, or pile onto a large share platter. Squeeze over the lemon juice, sprinkle over the lemon zest and top with dollops of the avocado dressing. Finish with the toasted pine nut and pumpkin seed crumb and serve.

GOOD TO KNOW: *This dish can be eaten cold or hot so feel free to make up a big batch. It will keep in an airtight container in the fridge for up to 7 days.*

HEALTH HACK: *Olives belong to a group of fruit called drupes, or stone fruits, and are related to mangoes, cherries, peaches, almonds and pistachios. An oily, salty, non-starchy fruit, they are a good source of vitamin E and other powerful antioxidants.*

SEA

FOOD

BARRAMUNDI LETTUCE CUPS

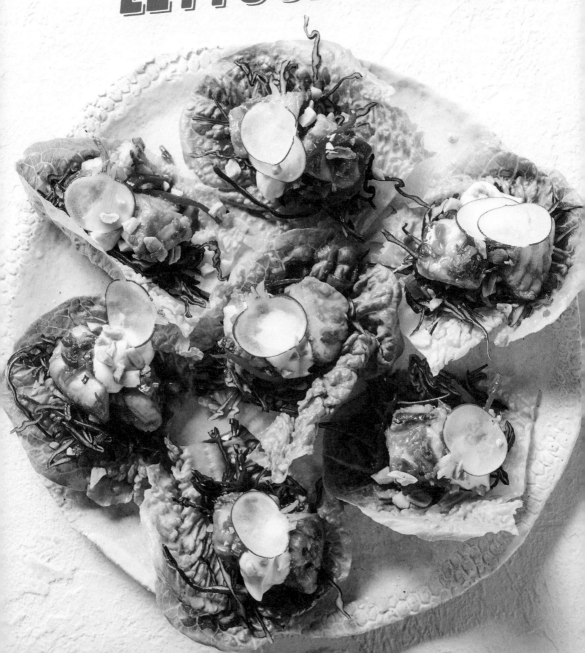

I ABSOLUTELY LOVE THE FRESHNESS THIS RECIPE BRINGS TO THE TABLE – THE WONDERFUL FLAVOURS OF THE FISH ALL WRAPPED UP IN THE LETTUCE CUPS, TOGETHER WITH THE CRUNCH FROM THE TOASTED PEANUTS, HELP MAKE IT A REAL CROWD FAVOURITE.

SERVES 4

2 tablespoons coconut oil
6 spring onions, finely sliced
1 long red chilli, deseeded and
   finely sliced
1 garlic clove, crushed
600 g barramundi or other firm white
   fish fillets, skin and bones removed,
   cut into 3 cm pieces
2 tablespoons tamari or
   coconut aminos
1 tablespoon sugar-free fish sauce
2 little gem lettuces, leaves separated
¼ red cabbage, finely shredded
4 radishes, finely sliced
Spicy Mayo (see page 86), to serve
2 tablespoons peanuts, crushed
   and toasted, to serve

Melt the coconut oil in a large frying pan over medium–high heat. Add the spring onion, chilli and garlic and saute for 1–2 minutes until slightly softened and caramelised. Add the fish pieces and cook, tossing, for 1–2 minutes or until they just start to colour on the edges. Stir through the tamari or coconut aminos and fish sauce, bring to a simmer and cook for a further 2–3 minutes, or until the sauce has reduced and thickened slightly.

To serve, arrange the lettuce leaves on a serving platter. Pile the fish mixture into the lettuce cups and top with the cabbage and radish slices. Finish each cup with a dollop of mayo and a scattering of peanuts – off you go!

GOOD TO KNOW: *When buying seafood, try to choose line-caught and sustainable where possible – doing so will help support ethical fishing practices and keep our oceans abundant with marine life for generations to come.*

HEALTH HACK: *When it comes to omega fatty acids, barramundi is both high in omega-3, which reduces inflammation, balances hormones and improves brain function, and low in omega-6, which is something you want to consume in moderation due to its inflammatory nature. Win-win, in other words!*

SALMON AND PUMPKIN FISHCAKES

SERVES 4

700 g butternut pumpkin, peeled
   and cut into 3 cm pieces
2 x 180 g salmon fillets, skin and
   bones removed
2 large handfuls of baby spinach leaves,
   roughly chopped
finely grated zest and juice of 1 lemon
100 g (1 cup) almond meal
3 tablespoons arrowroot or
   tapioca flour
1 egg, beaten
sea salt and freshly ground
   black pepper
3 tablespoons coconut oil

HERBED YOGHURT

250 g (1 cup) coconut yoghurt
1 tablespoon finely chopped dill
1 tablespoon finely chopped flat-leaf
   parsley leaves
finely grated zest and juice of 1 lemon

TO SERVE

1 lemon, sliced into wedges (optional)
1 handful of watercress leaves
8 cornichons, sliced lengthways

To make the herbed yoghurt, mix all the ingredients in a bowl. Transfer to the fridge to chill until needed.

Bring a saucepan of water to the boil over medium heat and place a steaming basket inside. Place the pumpkin into the steaming basket and cook for 8–10 minutes or until soft enough to press with a fork. Remove the pumpkin from the steamer basket and set aside.

Place the salmon in the steamer basket and cook for 3–4 minutes, or until the fillets are light pink on the outside and are almost cooked through. Remove from the heat and allow to cool.

Once the salmon has cooled, break it up into large flakes. Transfer to a bowl with the pumpkin, spinach, lemon zest and juice, almond meal, arrowroot or tapioca flour and egg, season with salt and pepper and gently fold together. Shape the mixture into 12 even-sized patties.

Melt the coconut oil in a large frying pan over medium–high heat. Working in two batches, cook the patties for 2–3 minutes on each side until lightly golden. Remove from the pan and set aside on paper towel to drain.

Divide the fishcakes among plates, season generously with salt and pepper and serve with the herbed yoghurt, lemon wedges (if using), watercress leaves and sliced cornichons.

GOOD TO KNOW: *This recipe is a good one to make in bulk for future use — simply freeze the fishcakes before cooking, then thaw as needed and cook as before. Once cooked they will keep in the fridge for up to 3 days.*

HEALTH HACK: *When we talk about the health benefits of salmon it's hard to go past its high omega-3 content. These long-chain omega-3 fatty acids can help reduce inflammation, lower blood pressure and decrease the risk factors for many diseases.*

YOU CAN'T GO PAST A GOOD FISHCAKE, AND THESE ONES ARE PARTICULARLY FLAVOURSOME AND EASY TO WHIP UP. WHILE THEY ARE GREAT AS THEY ARE, TO TAKE THEM TO THE NEXT LEVEL TRY STACKING THEM WITH YOUR FAVOURITE SALAD INGREDIENTS TO TRANSFORM THEM INTO BEAUTIFUL FISH BURGERS.

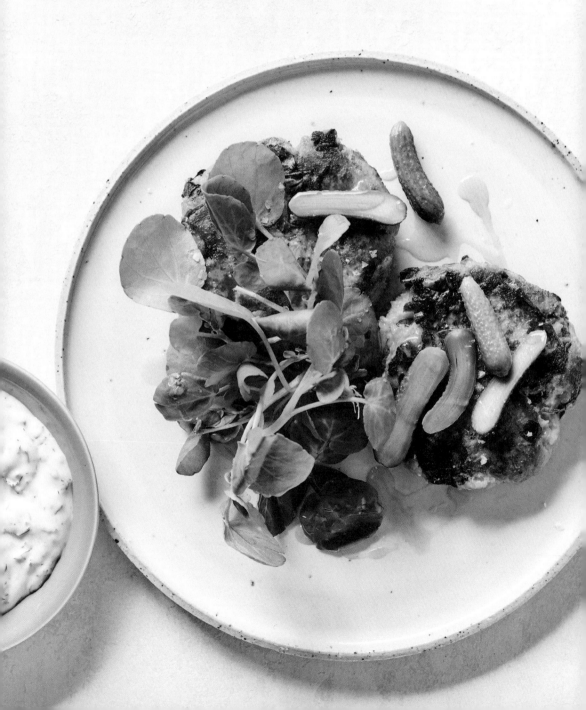

GORGEOUS GREEN FISH PARCELS

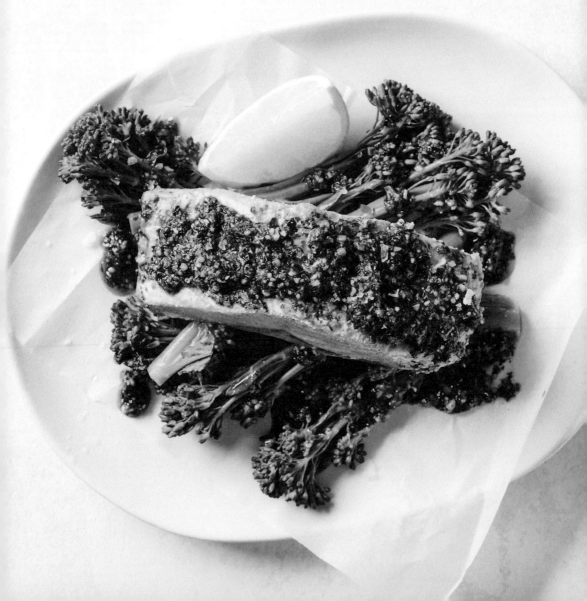

THIS RECIPE IS A SIMPLE YET DELICIOUSLY DIFFERENT WAY TO COOK YOUR FISH AND GREENS. COOKING EVERYTHING IN A PARCEL REALLY INTENSIFIES THE FLAVOURS AND HELPS TO MAKE EACH INGREDIENT SING.

SERVES 2

1 bunch of broccolini, trimmed
2 x 200 g ocean trout fillets, skin on
    and bones removed
2 tablespoons olive oil
juice of 1 lemon
sea salt and freshly ground
    black pepper
lemon wedges, to serve

PINE NUT PESTO

3 tablespoons extra-virgin olive oil
3 tablespoons pine nuts, toasted
1 handful of basil leaves
1 garlic clove, very finely chopped
finely grated zest and juice of 1 lemon
½ teaspoon sea salt

Preheat the oven to 200°C.

To make the pesto, place all the ingredients in a small food processor and pulse until just combined and still a little bit chunky. Set aside.

Lay a piece of foil about 50 cm in length on your work surface and fold it in half lengthways to form a double layer, then line with baking paper. Repeat with a second piece of foil.

Bring a saucepan of water to the boil, add the broccolini and blanch for 2 minutes. Transfer to a bowl of iced or very cold water and leave for 2 minutes. Drain, then divide the broccolini between the foil pieces.

Lay one of the ocean trout fillets, skin-side down, on top of the broccolini on one of the foil pieces and spoon over 1 tablespoon of the pesto. Drizzle over 1 tablespoon of olive oil, squeeze over half a lemon and season with salt and pepper. Repeat with the remaining ocean trout fillet.

Pull up the foil edges on each piece and scrunch them together to create two sealed parcels. Place your parcels on a baking tray and bake for 15 minutes. Remove the tray from the oven and leave to stand for 5 minutes, then carefully open each parcel – be careful of the steam! Carefully cut into each fillet to check they're cooked (if they aren't, simply rewrap and return to the oven for a minute or two longer), then slide onto plates and serve with the rest of the pesto and lemon wedges.

GOOD TO KNOW: *If you can't find good-quality ocean trout, simply sub it out for salmon or mackerel, or try this with any of your favourite white fish fillets – it'll still be delicious.*

HEALTH HACK: *A traditional pesto contains parmesan but, as you know, apart from grass-fed butter the majority of my recipes are dairy free. My rule with dairy is that it should always be full fat, from grass-fed cows and free-range animals eating a diet they were designed to eat in order to produce the most nutritious and best-quality product possible.*

SIMPLE CEVICHE with **AVOCADO CREAM** and **SALSA**

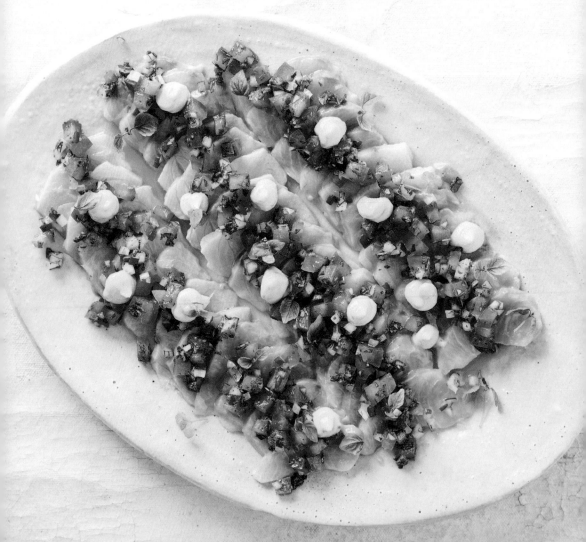

THIS IS A PERFECT SUMMER RECIPE WHEN YOU'RE LOOKING FOR SOMETHING QUICK AND EASY TO BRING TO THE TABLE. MOST ELEMENTS IN THIS DISH DON'T REQUIRE ANY COOKING, MEANING IT'S SUPER SIMPLE TO PUT TOGETHER — ALL YOU HAVE TO DO IS GET YOUR HANDS ON SOME WONDERFULLY FRESH FISH!

SERVES 4

540 g kingfish or other firm white fish
   fillets, skin off, bones removed and
   finely sliced
finely grated zest and juice of 3 limes
2 teaspoons tabasco sauce
1 teaspoon fine coconut sugar
2 tablespoons finely chopped chives

AVOCADO CREAM

2 avocados
2 tablespoons canned coconut cream
2 teaspoons extra-virgin olive oil
finely grated zest and juice of 1 lime
sea salt and freshly ground
   black pepper

TOMATO SALSA

4 tomatoes, deseeded, finely diced
½ red onion, finely diced
1 bunch of coriander, leaves
   roughly chopped
1 long red chilli, finely chopped
finely grated zest and juice of 1 lime
2 tablespoons extra-virgin olive oil
sea salt and freshly ground
   black pepper

TO SERVE

1 tablespoon extra-virgin olive oil
2 tablespoons finely chopped
   coriander leaves
2 tablespoons shredded coconut,
   toasted (optional)

Place the fish pieces, lime zest and juice, tabasco and coconut sugar in a bowl and mix well. Cover, transfer to the fridge and leave to chill for 30 minutes.

To make the avocado cream, whiz the avocado, coconut cream, oil, lemon zest and juice in a food processor until smooth. Season to taste with salt and pepper, cover and leave to chill in the fridge until needed.

For the tomato salsa, combine all the ingredients in a bowl. Set aside for 10 minutes to allow the flavours to develop.

To serve, drain the fish pieces and arrange them on individual plates or on a large serving platter. Dollop over spoonfuls of the tomato salsa and avocado cream, drizzle with a little extra-virgin olive oil and sprinkle over some finely chopped coriander leaves and toasted shredded coconut, if you like.

GOOD TO KNOW: *Originating in Peru, ceviche is typically made from fresh raw fish cured in citrus juices, such as lemon or lime, spiced with chilli peppers or other seasonings including chopped onion, salt and coriander. The key to making it is to ensure the fish is impeccably fresh, so be sure to ask your fishmonger when the fish was caught so you know what you're buying.*

HEALTH HACK: *Some research suggests that eating raw fish is particularly good for you, as it retains certain nutrients that are typically lost during the cooking process.*

SPICY COCONUT FISH BITES

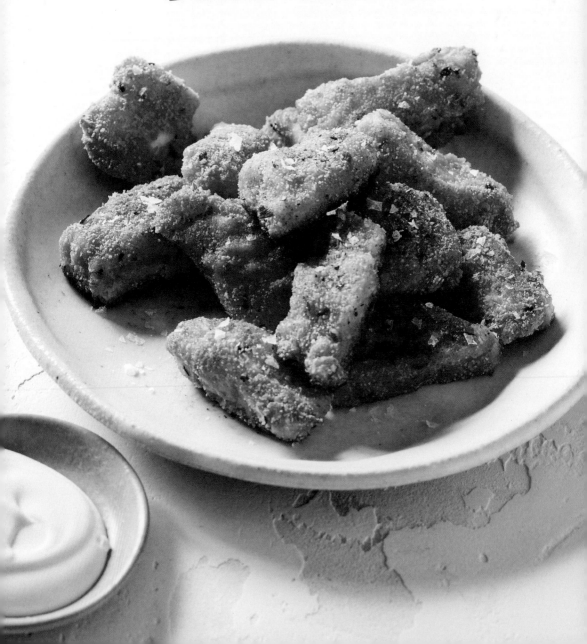

THIS IS A FANTASTIC DISH THAT EVERYONE WILL LOVE. THE COMBINATION OF CHILLI FLAKES AND CAYENNE PEPPER REALLY GIVE THESE LITTLE BITES A FIERY KICK.

SERVES 4

60 g (½ cup) arrowroot or
    tapioca flour
2 eggs, beaten
100 g (1 cup) almond meal
45 g (½ cup) desiccated coconut
½ teaspoon sea salt
1 teaspoon dried chilli flakes
½ teaspoon cayenne pepper
½ teaspoon sweet paprika
400 g whiting, snapper or other firm
    white fish fillets, skin off and bones
    removed, cut into 5 cm chunks
coconut oil spray
lemon wedges, to serve (optional)
Spicy Mayo (see page 86), to serve

Preheat the oven to 180°C and line a baking tray with baking paper.

Put the arrowroot or tapioca flour in one bowl, the egg in another, and the almond meal, desiccated coconut, salt, chilli, cayenne and paprika in a third bowl.

Dip the fish pieces into the arrowroot or tapioca flour, then the egg, allowing the excess to drip off, and finally into the almond and coconut mixture to coat well on all sides. Transfer the fish to the prepared tray and lightly spray with coconut oil. Bake for 10–12 minutes, turning halfway and re-spraying with oil if you wish, until golden brown and crisp.

Serve the fish bites with lemon wedges (if desired) and a bowl of mayo for dipping.

GOOD TO KNOW: *To give these more of a mild spice hit, try replacing the dried chilli flakes and cayenne pepper with some ground cumin and turmeric.*

HEALTH HACK: *Coconut meat is the white flesh of coconuts and is edible fresh or dried. This recipe celebrates it in its dried form as desiccated coconut. It is both rich in fibre and healthy fats, so it keeps you feeling fuller for longer.*

FIERY FISH CURRY
with CAULIFLOWER RICE

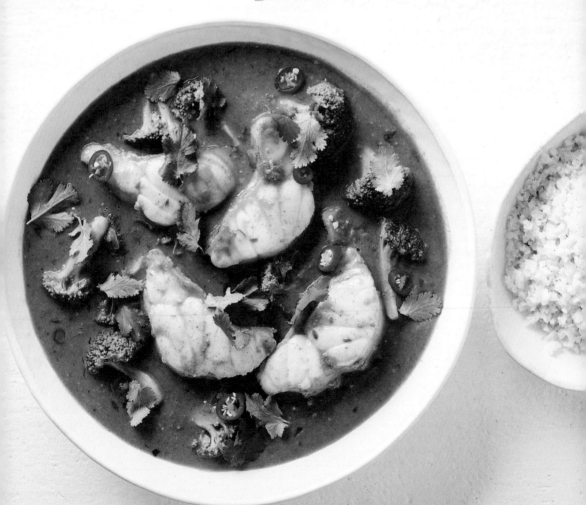

I WOULD HAVE TO SAY A HOME-COOKED CURRY TOPS MY LIST OF FAVOURITE MEALS. YOU'LL SEE I HAVE USED BARRAMUNDI HERE, THOUGH ANY FIRM WHITE FISH WORKS WELL, AND IT IS GREAT WITH CHICKEN THIGHS, TOO. MAKING THE CURRY PASTE IS PRETTY SIMPLE ONCE YOU'VE LEARNED HOW. GO ON, GIVE IT A TRY — I PROMISE YOU WON'T BE DISAPPOINTED WITH THE RESULTS!

SERVES 4

1 tablespoon coconut oil
1 red onion, roughly chopped
1 bunch of coriander, leaves separated
   and stems finely chopped
400 ml can coconut cream
500 ml (2 cups) chicken or fish stock
1 head of broccoli, broken into florets
4 x 150 g barramundi or other firm
   white fish fillets, skin and
   bones removed

CURRY PASTE

3 tablespoons desiccated coconut
5 cm piece of ginger, peeled and
   roughly chopped
4 garlic cloves, roughly chopped
1 tablespoon garam masala
1 tablespoon fennel seeds
1 tablespoon ground turmeric
1 teaspoon ground coriander
1 teaspoon ground cumin
1 long red chilli, deseeded and chopped
1 tablespoon sugar-free fish sauce
1 tablespoon coconut oil, melted
½ teaspoon sea salt
1–2 tablespoons boiling water (optional)

CAULIFLOWER RICE

1 head of cauliflower, florets
   and stalk roughly chopped
2 tablespoons coconut oil
sea salt

TO SERVE

1 handful of coriander leaves, torn
1 long red chilli, finely sliced
1 lime, sliced into wedges (optional)

To make the curry paste, place all the ingredients in a small food processor and blitz to form a paste (if it's too thick, add a dash of boiling water to loosen it up). Set aside.

For the cauliflower rice, place the chopped cauliflower in a food processor and pulse into tiny rice-like pieces (this usually takes six to eight pulses). Melt the coconut oil in a large frying pan over medium heat, add the cauliflower rice and saute for 4–6 minutes, or until softened. Season to taste with salt and keep warm.

Melt the coconut oil in a large deep frying pan or saucepan over medium–high heat. Add the onion and coriander stems and saute for 2–3 minutes until fragrant, then add the curry paste and fry for 4–5 minutes, stirring as you go, until aromatic. Pour over the coconut cream and stock and bring to the boil, then reduce the heat to low and simmer for 5 minutes to thicken and reduce slightly.

Add the broccoli florets to the pan and cook for 2–3 minutes, then lower the fish pieces into the curry and cook for 6–8 minutes or until the fish is just cooked.

Serve the curry with warm cauliflower rice, scattered with the coriander leaves, chilli and a squeeze of lime juice, if using.

GOOD TO KNOW: *Take note that the cooking time of the fish can vary depending on the size and thickness of your pieces, which is why it is a good idea to have them all a similar size.*

HEALTH HACK: *One of the things I love about this recipe is the fact it uses an easy homemade curry paste. This hands down beats any store-bought versions which can often contain hidden nasties like processed and refined sugars and inflammatory oils.*

HERBY FRIED FISH AND CHIPS

SERVES 4

2 eggs
3 tablespoons canned coconut cream
300 g (3 cups) almond meal
60 g (½ cup) arrowroot or
    tapioca flour
finely grated zest of 2 lemons
1 bunch of flat-leaf parsley, leaves
    finely chopped
2 teaspoons dried chilli flakes
½ teaspoon sea salt
4 × 125 g barramundi or other firm
    white fish fillets, skin and
    bones removed
2 avocados, each cut lengthways into
    6–8 wedges
2 zucchini, cut into long wedges
coconut, macadamia or avocado
    oil spray
125 ml (½ cup) coconut oil
mixed salad leaves, to serve
lemon wedges, to serve

Preheat the oven to 220°C and line a large baking tray with baking paper.

Whisk the eggs and coconut cream in a large shallow bowl.

In a separate bowl, combine the almond meal, arrowroot or tapioca flour, lemon zest, parsley, chilli flakes and salt.

Working with one piece at a time, dip the fish in the egg mixture, allowing excess liquid to drip off, then coat in the almond meal mixture before transferring to a plate. Refrigerate for 10 minutes.

Repeat the dipping and coating process with the avocado and zucchini wedges, arranging them evenly across the prepared baking tray and making sure there is space between each. Spray the avocado and zucchini generously with oil, then bake for 15–20 minutes or until crispy and golden brown.

While the 'chips' are cooking, heat the coconut oil in a large non-stick frying pan over medium–high heat until the oil is shimmering. Carefully lower the fish pieces into the oil and shallow-fry for 2–3 minutes on each side, or until golden and crisp. Transfer to paper towel to drain off any excess oil.

Divide the fish and 'chips' among plates, season generously with salt and serve with salad leaves and lemon wedges.

GOOD TO KNOW: *Feel free to mix up the fresh herbs to suit your taste. Both coriander and mint work well with (or in place of) the flat-leaf parsley.*

HEALTH HACK: *You'll notice that whenever I shallow-fry anything in my recipes I use coconut oil. This is because it has a high smoke point, meaning it is stable at higher temperatures and doesn't lose any of its nutritional properties during the cooking process.*

MY ULTIMATE CHEAT MEAL IS BEER-BATTERED FISH AND CHIPS — I JUST LOVE THE FLAVOURS AND TEXTURES. THIS HEALTHIER VERSION MEANS THAT EVERYONE (MYSELF INCLUDED!) DOING THE KICKSTART CAN STILL INDULGE, BUT WITH ALL THE ADDED AWESOMENESS THAT COMES FROM USING GOOD-QUALITY INGREDIENTS.

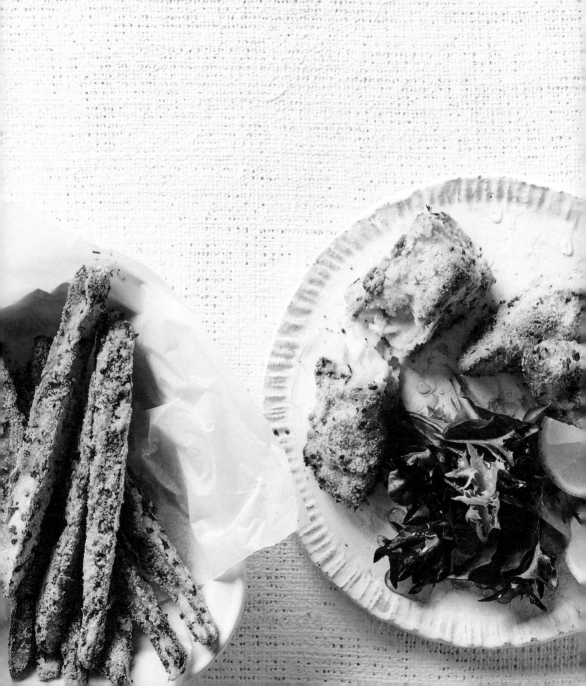

ZINGY FISH TACOS WITH SMASHED AVO

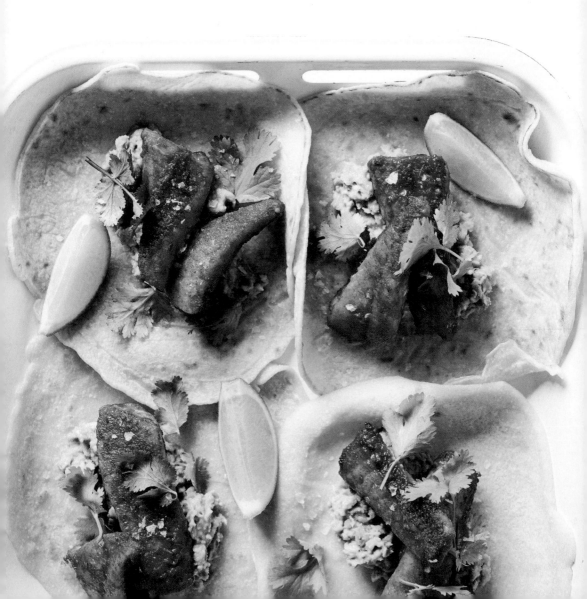

I LOVE A GOOD TACO, AND THIS ONE IS BASED ON THE CLASSIC BAJA FISH TACO OF MEXICAN AND SOUTHERN CALIFORNIAN FAME. THE SOFT COCONUT TORTILLAS ARE REALLY EASY TO MAKE AND SUPER VERSATILE — GIVE THEM A TRY AND YOU'LL SOON BE WHIPPING THEM UP TO GO WITH CHILLIS, SKEWERS AND ... WELL, PRETTY MUCH EVERYTHING!

SERVES 4

400 g snapper or other firm white
   fish fillets, skin and bones removed
2 tablespoons extra-virgin olive oil
1 tablespoon arrowroot or
   tapioca flour
1 tablespoon smoked paprika
2 teaspoons ground cumin
½ teaspoon cayenne pepper
1 teaspoon sea salt
½ teaspoon freshly ground
   black pepper
1 teaspoon garlic powder
1 teaspoon dried thyme
3 tablespoons coconut oil

COCONUT TORTILLAS

2 large eggs, beaten
250 ml (1 cup) canned coconut milk
125 g (1 cup) arrowroot or
   tapioca flour
3 tablespoons coconut flour
½ teaspoon sea salt
2 tablespoons extra-virgin olive oil

TO SERVE

2 avocados, roughly smashed with
   a fork
1 handful of coriander leaves,
   roughly torn
1 lime, cut into wedges

To make the coconut tortillas, whisk all the ingredients except the oil in a bowl to form a smooth batter. Heat a little of the oil in a frying pan over medium heat. Pour 3 tablespoons of the batter into the pan, then tilt and swirl the pan to spread the batter into a 15 cm circle. Reduce the heat to low and cook for 1–2 minutes until sturdy enough to flip, then cook for 1–2 minutes on the other side until cooked through, puffed up and golden brown. Transfer the tortilla to a plate and repeat this process, adding a little more oil each time, to make eight tortillas. Wrap in a tea towel to keep warm while you prepare the fish.

Cut the fish fillets into smaller pieces about 8 cm in length, place in a bowl and drizzle over the extra-virgin olive oil. In a separate bowl combine the arrowroot or tapioca flour, spices, salt, pepper, garlic powder and dried thyme. Sprinkle the dry spice mix over the fish and toss to coat well.

Melt the coconut oil in a large non-stick frying pan over medium–high heat. Add the coated fish pieces and fry for 2–3 minutes on each side, or until golden brown and cooked through.

To serve, spoon a little smashed avo over the middle of a warm tortilla, top with a few fish pieces and scatter over some coriander leaves. Give everything a good squeeze of fresh lime juice, season well with salt and enjoy.

GOOD TO KNOW: *Instead of eight smaller soft tacos, feel free to make four larger ones by pouring 125 ml (½ cup) of batter into the pan. As the tortillas will be slightly thicker, allow an extra 30–60 seconds of cooking time for each side.*

HEALTH HACK: *Store-bought tortillas often contain gluten and are high in carbohydrates, unlike these delicious homemade ones, which are a fantastic option for keeping you on track during your kickstart and beyond.*

CHIC

BKEN

CRISPY BUTTER CHICKEN SALAD

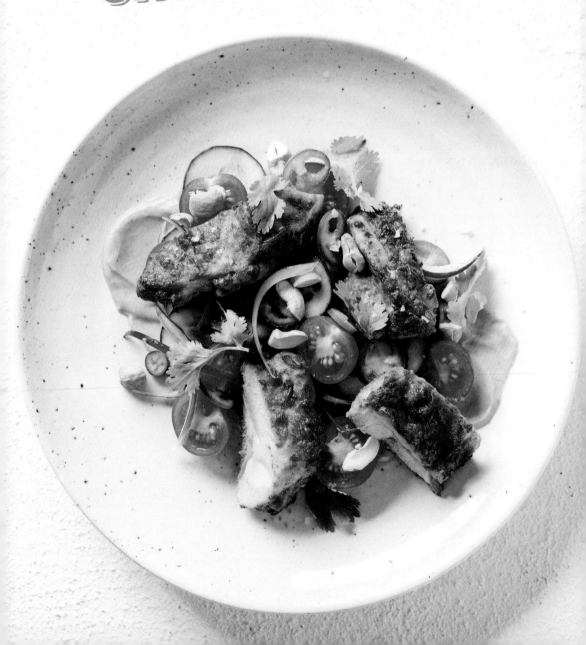

I AM A MASSIVE FAN OF BUTTER CHICKEN. HERE I WANTED TO SHOW YOU A DIFFERENT WAY TO EAT IT, TURNING IT INTO A LUSCIOUS SALAD STUFFED FULL OF ALL THE FLAVOURS YOU KNOW AND LOVE, BUT ALSO BURSTING WITH AN EXTRA LEVEL OF FRESHNESS.

SERVES 4

1 tablespoon extra-virgin olive oil
2 teaspoons garam masala
250 g (1 cup) coconut yoghurt
6 chicken thighs, skin on
1 Lebanese cucumber, sliced into
    rounds
250 g truss tomatoes, halved
2 green chillies, finely sliced
1 red onion, finely sliced
1 handful of coriander leaves
1 tablespoon apple cider vinegar
pinch of sea salt
finely grated zest and juice of 1 lime
80 g (½ cup) cashew nuts, toasted
    and chopped

TANDOORI PASTE

1 tablespoon coconut oil, melted
1 teaspoon ground ginger
1 teaspoon ground cumin
1 teaspoon ground coriander
1 teaspoon ground turmeric
1 teaspoon smoked paprika
1 teaspoon cayenne pepper
1 teaspoon sea salt

To make the tandoori paste, mix all the ingredients in a small bowl. Set aside.

In a large bowl, mix the olive oil, garam masala, half the coconut yoghurt and two-thirds of the tandoori paste. Add the chicken thighs and toss to coat in the marinade, then set aside for 15–20 minutes to absorb all the yummy flavours.

Preheat the oven to 180°C and line a baking tray with baking paper.

Arrange the chicken thighs skin-side up on the prepared tray. Bake for 10–12 minutes, or until cooked through and golden brown and crispy on top.

Meanwhile, combine the cucumber, tomato, green chilli, red onion and coriander in a bowl. Add the apple cider vinegar, salt and lime zest and juice, and toss to coat well.

In a separate bowl, mix the remaining coconut yoghurt and tandoori paste.

When ready to serve, spread the yoghurt and tandoori mixture across your serving plates and pile the fresh, zesty salad ingredients on top. Slice the chicken thighs into thick strips and lay these on top of the salad, then scatter over the cashews and season with salt. Enjoy!

GOOD TO KNOW: *For really lovely charred chicken skin, try switching the oven over to the grill function for the last few minutes of cooking time. You could also thread the chicken onto skewers, if preferred.*

HEALTH HACK: *The reason I want you to make your own tandoori paste is that most store-bought versions contain refined sugars, inflammatory seed oils, and artificial colours and flavours. It's always best to stick with real food.*

CHARRED COCONUT CHICKEN SKEWERS

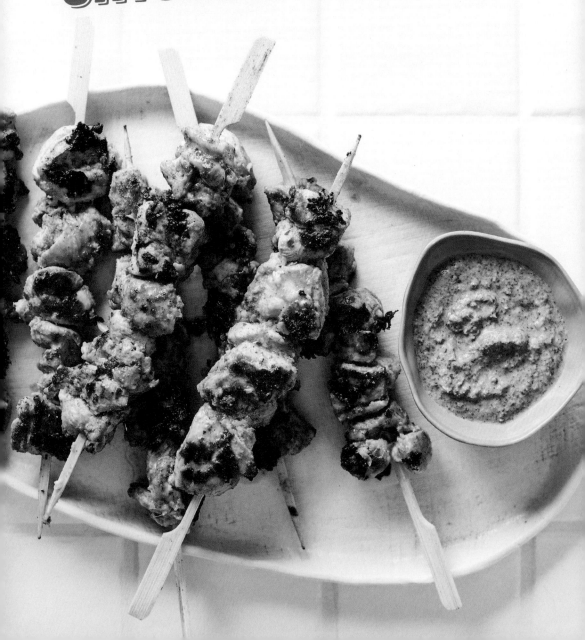

I AM ALL ABOUT TEXTURES WHEN IT COMES TO COOKING, WHICH IS WHY I LOVE ALL THINGS CRISPY, CRUNCHY OR, IN THIS CASE, CHARRED. DIFFERENT COOKING METHODS PRODUCE DIFFERENT FLAVOURS, AND WHEN IT COMES TO CHICKEN, CHARRING IT GIVES IT A SMOKY, CARAMELISED FLAVOUR THAT IS PRETTY MUCH IMPOSSIBLE TO RESIST.

SERVES 4

800 g chicken thighs, cut into
   3 cm chunks
250 ml (1 cup) canned coconut cream
finely grated zest and juice of 1 lime
5 cm piece of ginger, peeled and
   finely grated
2 garlic cloves, very finely chopped
2 teaspoons ground turmeric
1 teaspoon dried chilli flakes
1 teaspoon ground cardamom
1 teaspoon ground cumin
1 tablespoon coconut oil, grass-fed
   butter or ghee, melted
2 tablespoons shredded coconut,
   toasted (optional)
1 green bird's eye chilli, finely
   sliced (optional)

SPICY SALSA

2 bunches of coriander, leaves picked
2 bunches of mint, leaves picked
1 long green chilli, roughly chopped
juice of 1½ limes
1 teaspoon ground coriander
2 tablespoons canned coconut cream
2 tablespoons extra-virgin olive,
   avocado or macadamia oil
sea salt and freshly ground
   black pepper

Place eight bamboo skewers in a shallow dish, cover with cold water and leave to soak for at least 30 minutes.

Place the chicken, coconut cream, lime zest and juice, ginger, garlic, turmeric, chilli, cardamom and cumin in a large bowl and combine. Cover, transfer to the fridge and marinate for at least 15 minutes, or up to 1 hour for best results.

While the chicken is marinating, make the salsa. Place all the ingredients in a food processor or high-speed blender and blitz until smooth. Set aside.

Heat a chargrill pan or barbecue grill to high.

Thread the marinated chicken pieces onto the prepared skewers and brush well with your chosen cooking fat. Grill the skewers for 3–4 minutes each side, or until cooked through and charred and golden brown on the outside.

Transfer the skewers to a serving platter. Sprinkle over the coconut and green chilli, if using, and serve with the salsa.

GOOD TO KNOW: *For those who don't have a barbecue, a chargrill pan or griddle pan can be found in most kitchenware stores. They are often square and are easily identifiable by the grill lines on the base, which help to create that lovely char line on food. The key to successful chargrilling on one of these pans is making sure you preheat them so they're nice and hot!*

HEALTH HACK: *You'll notice that across my recipes in this book, when I call for coconut milk or cream, I specify it should be from a can. The reason for this is that a number of the carton-packed versions contain sugars, oils, thickeners or fillers.*

CRISPY CAYENNE CHICKEN WITH SIMPLE SALSA

SERVES 4

3 tablespoons extra-virgin olive, avocado or macadamia oil
2 teaspoons smoked paprika
1 teaspoon cayenne pepper
1 teaspoon ground cumin
2 garlic cloves, very finely chopped
800 g chicken thighs, skin on
2 avocados
freshly grated zest and juice of 1 lemon
sea salt and freshly ground black pepper
2 limes, halved
Tomato Salsa (see page 103), to serve
microherbs, to serve (optional)

Combine your chosen oil with the paprika, cayenne pepper, cumin and garlic in a bowl. Add the chicken thighs and coat well. Cover, transfer to the fridge and leave to marinate for at least 10 minutes, or up to 1 hour for best results.

Place the avocado in a bowl, mash roughly with a fork and mix well with the lemon zest and juice. Season well with salt and set aside.

Heat a chargrill pan or barbecue grill to high.

Grill the chicken thighs for 4 minutes before turning. Add the limes cut-side down to the grill and cook for another 4 minutes, or until the lime flesh is charred, the chicken is cooked through and the skin is charred, crispy and crunchy.

Cut the chicken thighs into thirds and serve with the salsa, generous dollops of the smashed avocado and the charred lime halves. Add some microherbs, if using, season well with salt and pepper and enjoy.

GOOD TO KNOW: *If you fancy mixing it up from time to time, this recipe also works well with pork fillets or loin.*

HEALTH HACK: *Studies show the capsaicin in cayenne peppers may help to reduce hunger, making you feel fuller for longer and reducing snacking.*

THIS DISH IS THE PERFECT EXAMPLE OF JUST HOW SIMPLE A GREAT MEAL CAN BE. ALL YOU HAVE TO DO IS TAKE ONE EVERYDAY PROTEIN, COAT IT IN DELICIOUS SPICES AND THROW IT TOGETHER WITH A SPEEDY SALSA THAT'S EXPLODING WITH FLAVOUR. WHAT MORE DO YOU NEED?

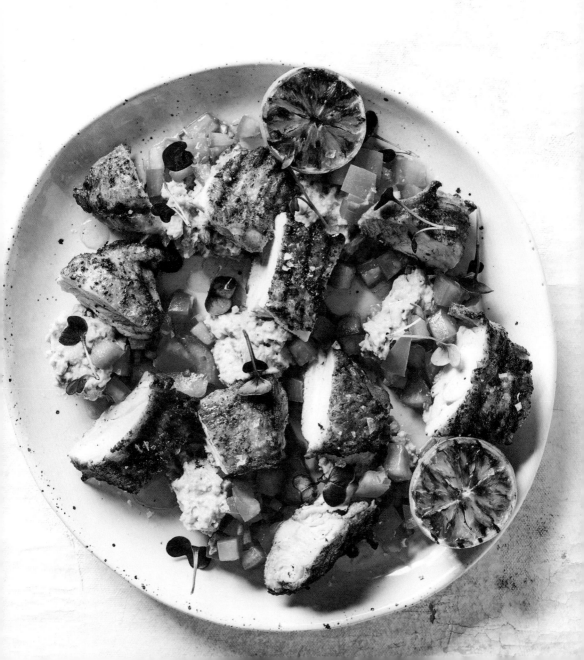

SIMPLE SATAY AND SLAW

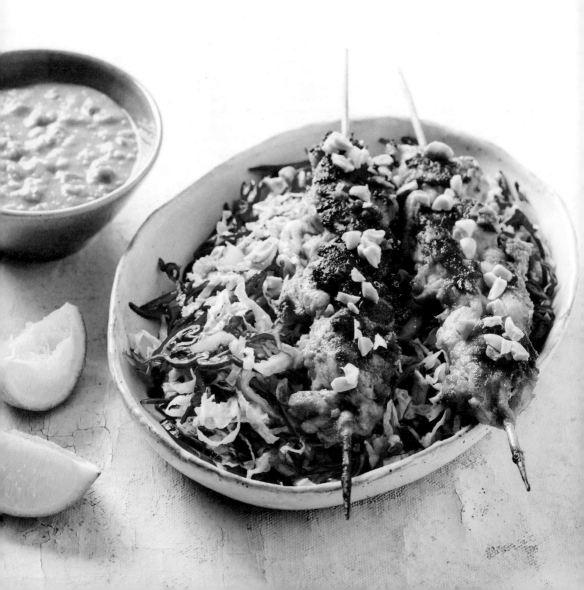

ACROSS MY BOOKS I'VE MADE A FEW DIFFERENT VERSIONS OF SATAY SAUCE, AND HERE'S A NEW TAKE ON AN OLD FAVOURITE. HERE I'VE USED TAMARIND, A FRUIT THAT MOST OFTEN APPEARS IN ASIAN AND MIDDLE EASTERN COOKING, TO GIVE A SLIGHTLY SOUR, TANGY FLAVOUR. IT CAN BE FOUND IN MOST SUPERMARKETS IN PASTE AND PUREE FORM. HUNT IT DOWN AND I PROMISE YOU WON'T BE DISAPPOINTED WITH THE RESULTS.

SERVES 4

800 g chicken thighs (about 8), halved
3 tablespoons peanuts, toasted and
    roughly chopped
lime wedges, to serve

SLAW
½ Chinese cabbage (wombok),
    finely shredded
¼ red cabbage, finely shredded
3 tablespoons sesame seeds, toasted
2 teaspoons extra-virgin olive,
    avocado or macadamia oil
finely grated zest and juice of 2 limes

SATAY SAUCE
2 tablespoons coconut oil
1 lemongrass stalk, inner core only
    (see Good to Know), finely chopped
2 garlic cloves, finely grated
5 cm piece of ginger, peeled and
    finely grated
½ red onion, finely chopped
½ teaspoon dried chilli flakes
2 teaspoons coconut sugar
2 teaspoons tamarind paste or puree
2 tablespoons tamari
125 g (½ cup) peanut butter
finely grated zest and juice of 1 lime
250 ml (1 cup) filtered water
sea salt

Place eight bamboo skewers in a shallow dish, cover with cold water and leave to soak for at least 30 minutes.

To make the slaw, toss the cabbage and sesame seeds in a bowl. Add the oil, lime zest and juice and toss again. Cover and set aside in the fridge until needed.

For the satay sauce, melt the coconut oil in a frying pan over medium heat. Add the lemongrass, garlic, ginger, onion and chilli flakes and cook, stirring, for 4–5 minutes or until the onion is softened and caramelised. Add the rest of the ingredients (except the salt) and cook, stirring, for 1–2 minutes until thickened slightly. Season to taste with salt, then remove from the heat and set aside to cool.

Heat a barbecue grill or chargrill pan to high.

Thread the chicken pieces onto the prepared skewers. Lightly brush the skewers all over with 80 ml (⅓ cup) of the satay sauce, then cook, turning regularly, for 8–10 minutes or until cooked through and charred and golden brown on the outside.

To serve, divide the slaw among plates or bowls. Top with the chicken skewers, drizzle with the remaining satay sauce and sprinkle over the chopped peanuts. Serve with lime wedges for squeezing.

GOOD TO KNOW: *When it comes to lemongrass, only the tender bottom third of each stalk is edible. To prepare, remove the tough outer leaves and pound with a rolling pin or the back of a knife.*

HEALTH HACK: *If you're strictly paleo and avoid legumes, simply replace the peanut butter and peanuts for almond butter and almonds.*

RAS-EL-HANOUT CHOOK WITH CHILLI AND LIME YOGHURT

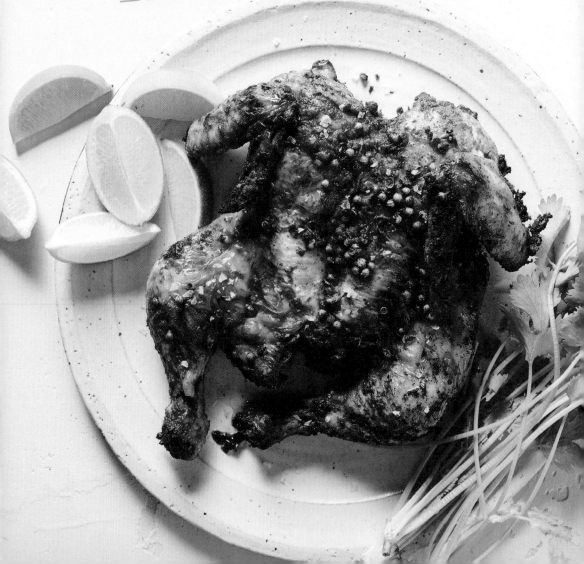

WITH ITS FLAVOURSOME SPICES, THIS IS ONE OF MY FAVOURITE WAYS TO CELEBRATE A ROAST CHOOK. RAS-EL-HANOUT IS A SPICE MIX FOUND IN VARYING FORMS IN TUNISIA, ALGERIA AND MOROCCO. THE NAME LITERALLY TRANSLATES TO 'HEAD OF THE SHOP' AND IMPLIES A MIX OF THE BEST SPICES THE SELLER HAS TO OFFER.

SERVES 4

250 g (1 cup) coconut yoghurt
sea salt
finely grated zest and juice of 1 lime
1.5 kg butterflied whole chicken
   (see Good to Know)
2 tablespoons extra-virgin olive oil
freshly ground black pepper
1 handful of coriander or flat-leaf
   parsley leaves, roughly torn
lime wedges, to serve

RAS-EL-HANOUT

1 tablespoon coriander seeds
2 teaspoons cumin seeds
2 teaspoons ground cinnamon
2 teaspoons smoked paprika
1 teaspoon dried chilli flakes
1 teaspoon ground cardamom
1 teaspoon ground ginger
1 teaspoon ground turmeric

To make the ras-el-hanout, place all the ingredients in a small food processor or high-speed blender and blitz to a rough powder. I like to leave it on the rougher side, with some of the seeds left whole.

Transfer the ras-el-hanout to a large bowl or a shallow glass baking dish. Add the coconut yoghurt, 1 teaspoon of salt, the lime zest and juice and mix well.

Using a sharp knife, cut two shallow slits in each of the chicken breasts and legs, then place the chicken in the marinade and turn to coat well. Set aside on the bench to marinate for 30 minutes.

Preheat a chargrill pan or barbecue grill to medium–high and the oven to 180°C. Line a baking tray with baking paper.

When ready to cook, remove the chicken from the marinade allowing any excess to drip off. Drizzle the olive oil over the chicken then transfer, breast-side down, to the hot pan or grill and cook for 10 minutes, turning halfway through, until golden brown and charred all over.

Transfer the chicken, breast-side up, to the prepared baking tray and roast in the oven for 30–40 minutes, or until the juices run clear when the thickest part of the thigh is pierced with a skewer. Remove from the oven, cover loosely with foil and leave to rest for 10 minutes.

When ready to serve, cut the chicken into pieces and season generously with salt and pepper. Top with the herbs and serve with lime wedges for squeezing.

GOOD TO KNOW: *I've called for a butterflied chook here as it results in a quicker, more even cook. Your local butcher will be able to do this for you on request but if for whatever reason you can't get your hands on a butterflied chook, simply follow this recipe with a regular one instead. Omit the chargrill pan process and slip it into the oven for 40–60 minutes, or until cooked through and the juices run clear when the thickest part of the thigh is pierced with a skewer.*

CHICKEN 'N' BACON WRAPS WITH ZESTY AVO SMASH

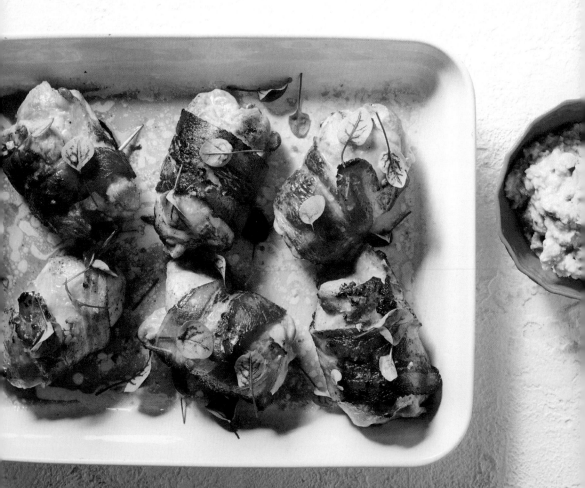

THERE IS SUCH A LOVELY SIMPLICITY TO THIS DISH – IT'S A RICH, FLAVOURSOME AND GENEROUS FEED THAT CAN BE SERVED STRAIGHT FROM THE PAN FOR EVERYONE TO ENJOY.

SERVES 4

3 tablespoons coconut oil, grass-fed
   butter or ghee, melted
1 teaspoon apple cider vinegar
finely grated zest and juice of 1 lemon
1 teaspoon mustard powder
½ teaspoon chilli powder
½ teaspoon smoked paprika
4 large or 8 small chicken thighs
4 or 8 streaky bacon rashers
1 handful of soft herbs, such as sorrel,
   coriander or parsley, leaves picked
sea salt and freshly ground
   black pepper

ZESTY AVO SMASH
1 avocado
finely grated zest and juice of 1 lime
1 tablespoon apple cider vinegar
1 teaspoon dried chilli flakes
sea salt

Preheat the oven to 180°C.

For the avo smash, scoop the avocado flesh into a bowl and gently mash it with the back of a fork. Mix in the rest of the ingredients, then set aside in the fridge until ready to serve.

In a bowl, whisk your preferred cooking fat, apple cider vinegar, lemon zest and juice, mustard powder, chilli powder and smoked paprika. Add the chicken thighs to the bowl and toss well to coat.

Lay out a bacon rasher on a chopping board and place one of the chicken thighs at one end. Roll up the rasher so that the bacon is tightly wrapped around the chicken, covering as much of it as possible, then secure with a toothpick. Repeat with the remaining chicken and bacon.

Heat a large ovenproof frying-pan over medium heat. Add the wrapped chicken thighs and fry for 3–4 minutes on each side, or until crispy and golden brown all over. Transfer to a baking dish and place in the oven to roast until cooked through (about 10–12 minutes for smaller thighs and up to 15 minutes for larger thighs).

Remove from the oven and set aside to rest for 5 minutes in the pan. Scatter over the herbs, season with salt and pepper and serve with dollops of the zesty avo smash.

GOOD TO KNOW: *One day, when I was feeling extra creative, I tried tucking a dollop of the avo smash in with each chicken thigh before wrapping them up in the bacon. You should totally try it some time!*

HEALTH HACK: *When choosing bacon, don't forget that we should only support free-range nitrate-free bacon from pigs that have lived a good life without any hormones or stalls.*

LUKE'S 'ZINGER' BURGER

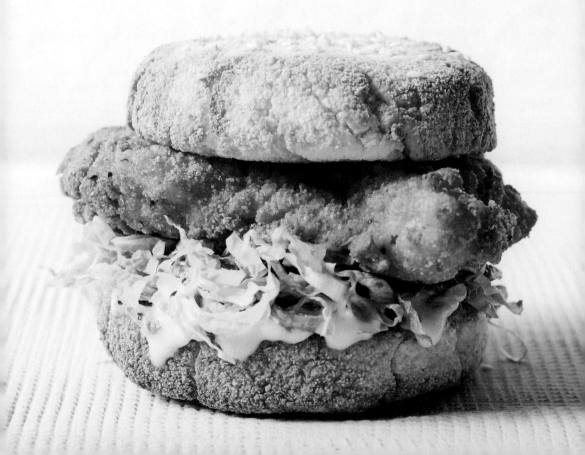

IF YOU LIKE IT HOT AND SPICY, MY 'ZINGER' BURGER WILL BE SURE TO HIT THE SPOT. THIS IS MY HEALTHIER TAKE ON THE FAST–FOOD FAVOURITE – THINK MOIST CHICKEN COATED IN CRUNCHY, SPICY SEASONING AND SERVED WITH CRISP LETTUCE AND CREAMY MAYO ON A SEEDED BUN. IT REALLY PACKS A PUNCH!

SERVES 4

60 g (½ cup) arrowroot or
    tapioca flour
150 g (1½ cups) almond meal
1 tablespoon dried chilli powder
1 teaspoon mustard powder
½ teaspoon dried chilli flakes
½ teaspoon sea salt, plus extra
    for seasoning
2 eggs
125 ml (½ cup) canned coconut milk
4 chicken thighs
coconut oil, for deep-frying

NO-FAIL PLANT-BASED MAYO

3 tablespoons extra-virgin olive
    or macadamia oil
3 tablespoons avocado or hemp
    seed oil
125 ml (½ cup) coconut oil, chilled
    until firm
2 teaspoons dijon mustard
½ teaspoon sea salt
2 tablespoons apple cider vinegar
juice of ½ lemon
1 tablespoon maple syrup or
    coconut nectar

TO SERVE

4 Bangin' Buns (see page 57)
½ cos lettuce, shredded

To make the mayo, in a high-speed blender or using a hand-held blender, blitz the oils, mustard, salt and vinegar until smooth. Add the lemon juice and sweetener of choice and blitz again until completely combined. Pour into a glass jar with a lid and transfer to the fridge until needed.

For the chicken, create a crumbing station of bowls. Put the arrowroot or tapioca flour in one bowl, mix the almond meal, spices and salt in another bowl, and in a third bowl whisk the eggs and coconut milk.

Working in batches of one or two, place the chicken thighs in the arrowroot flour and coat well, then dip them in the egg mixture, allowing any extra egg to drip off before finally coating them in the almond meal mixture. Transfer to a plate.

Half-fill a large, heavy-based saucepan with coconut oil and set over medium–high heat. Heat the oil to 160°C. To test if it is hot enough, simply place the end of a wooden spoon into the oil in the centre of the saucepan – if bubbles start to rise, you're good to go.

Working in two batches, carefully lower the chicken into the hot oil. Fry for 5–6 minutes, turning halfway through, until crispy and cooked through. Remove from the pan and drain on paper towel. Season with salt.

To construct your zingers, split the buns and smear a generous amount of mayo over the base of each, then pile on the lettuce followed by the crispy, chunky chicken. Sandwich the burgers together with the bun lids and devour.

GOOD TO KNOW: *If you don't want to make the rolls, simply use store-bought low-carb buns or serve these in lettuce cups instead. Feel like you need more vegetables? No worries – add some sliced tomatoes and red onion!*

HEALTH HACK: *When people 'go clean' with their diet they often think they'll have to miss out on all their favourite take-away foods, but this is not the case! This recipe, for example, hits the spot without any seed oils, refined sugars, colours, thickeners, flavours or gluten, so you can tuck in without the worry!*

CHICKEN CURRY MUFFINS

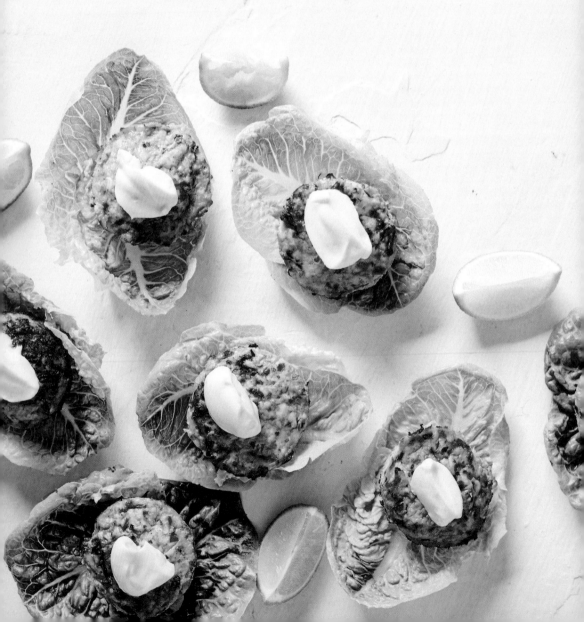

I HAVE ALWAYS SAID SPICES ARE YOUR BEST FRIEND IN THE KITCHEN, AND THESE AWESOME LITTLE MUFFINS PROVE IT. THIS HAS GOT TO BE ONE OF THE QUICKEST AND SIMPLEST RECIPES I HAVE EVER CREATED. REST ASSURED — WHAT IT LACKS IN EFFORT OR TIME IT CERTAINLY MAKES UP FOR IN FLAVOUR AND NUTRITION.

SERVES 4

2 tablespoons coconut oil, grass-fed butter or ghee, plus extra for greasing
2 garlic cloves, very finely chopped
1 long red chilli, finely chopped
1 red onion, finely chopped
600 g chicken mince
1 egg
1 zucchini, coarsely grated
60 g (½ cup) grated pumpkin
1 handful of flat-leaf parsley leaves, finely chopped
3 teaspoons curry powder (see Good to Know)
1 tablespoon coconut aminos
3 tablespoons chicken bone broth or 2 tablespoons powdered bone broth
sea salt and freshly ground black pepper

TO SERVE

2 baby gem lettuces, leaves separated
3 tablespoons No-fail Plant-based Mayo (see page 127) (optional)
1 lime, cut into wedges

Preheat the oven to 180°C and lightly grease a regular 12-hole muffin tray with your preferred cooking fat.

Heat your preferred cooking fat in a large frying pan over medium heat. Add the garlic, chilli and onion and saute for 4–5 minutes, until softened and caramelised. Remove from the heat and set aside.

In a bowl, mix the chicken, egg, zucchini, pumpkin, parsley, curry powder, coconut aminos, broth and onion mixture. Season with salt and pepper, then spoon the mixture evenly into the prepared muffin tray.

Bake for 12–15 minutes until cooked through and golden brown on top. Remove from the oven and set the muffins aside to cool slightly in the tin.

To serve, pile lettuce leaves up one inside the other to create lettuce cups. Place a chicken muffin in the centre of each cup and top with a generous dollop of mayo, if you like. Squeeze over a little lime.

GOOD TO KNOW: *Finding a good curry powder is really easy now that there are heaps of great 'real' versions available at leading supermarkets and health food stores, so get out there, read your labels and choose one with the right taste and heat level for you. My favourite store-bought version contains only 100% natural ingredients and is made from a blend of nine different spices. Yum!*

HEALTH HACK: *To make this meal a little more filling, try swapping out the less energy-dense chicken for a higher-fat alternative such as beef or lamb mince.*

CRUNCHY APPLE AND CHICKEN SALAD

SERVES 4

4 chicken thighs, skin on
sea salt and freshly ground
   black pepper
2 tablespoons coconut oil, grass-fed
   butter or ghee
½ savoy cabbage, finely shredded
¼ red cabbage, finely shredded
½ red onion, finely sliced
1 green apple, cored and cut into
   matchsticks
1 handful of mint leaves, roughly torn
1 handful of flat-leaf parsley leaves,
   roughly torn
100 g (1 cup) pecans, toasted and
   roughly chopped

AVOCADO DRESSING

1 avocado
3 tablespoons extra-virgin olive oil
1 tablespoon apple cider vinegar
finely grated zest and juice of
   ½ lemon
sea salt and freshly ground
   black pepper

Pat the chicken pieces dry with paper towel and season the skin generously with salt.

Heat your preferred cooking fat in a large heavy-based frying pan over medium–high heat. Place the chicken thighs into the pan, skin-side down, and fry undisturbed for 7–8 minutes, or until the skin has rendered down and is golden brown and crispy. Flip over and cook for a further 3–4 minutes, or until completely cooked through. Transfer to paper towel to drain off any excess fat and leave to cool, then cut into thick strips.

To make the dressing, scoop the avocado flesh into a bowl and roughly mash it with a fork, then add the remaining ingredients and whisk until thick and creamy.

When you are ready to serve, place the shredded cabbage, onion, apple, herbs and pecans in a large bowl and toss well. Spread the salad across a serving platter, top with the chicken pieces and dollop over the avocado dressing. Season with salt and pepper and dig in!

GOOD TO KNOW: *This salad is a great, simple base and is really versatile, so feel free to swap out the chicken for any of your other favourite proteins.*

HEALTH HACK: *Apples are a fantastic source of fibre, which keeps us feeling fuller for longer (and helps us get us through our fasts).*

THIS SALAD IS MY SUBTLE NOD TO THE AWESOME FLAVOURS IN A CLASSIC WALDORF SALAD. I HAVE ALWAYS LOVED APPLES IN SALADS, AND THE CREAMINESS OF THE AVOCADO DRESSING REALLY TAKES THIS ONE TO THE NEXT LEVEL.

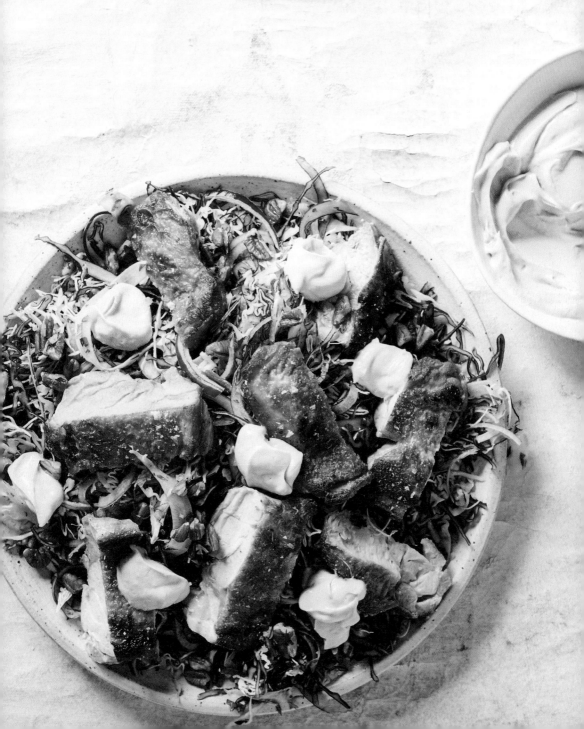

JERK DRUMSTICKS with ZESTY LIME CAULIFLOWER SMASH

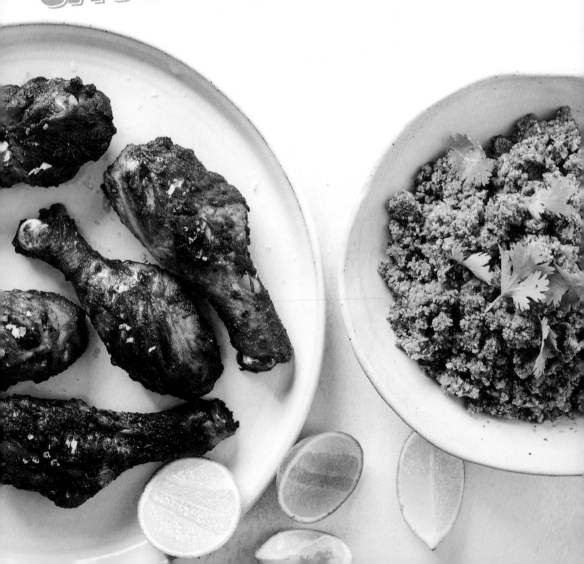

I THINK DRUMSTICKS ARE ONE OF THE MOST UNDERRATED CUTS OF CHICKEN. WHILE IT'S TRUE THAT, AS A COOK, I TEND TO FAVOUR THIGHS OR BREAST, THIS RECIPE IS AN EXCELLENT REMINDER OF HOW GREAT A DRUMSTICK CAN BE. THE JERK SPICE MIX HERE IS MY TAKE ON THE JAMAICAN CLASSIC — IT'S A REAL TASTEBUD TINGLER.

SERVES 4

3 tablespoons extra-virgin olive, avocado or macadamia oil
finely grated zest and juice of 1 lemon
sea salt and freshly ground black pepper
8 chicken drumsticks
1 handful of coriander leaves, roughly chopped
lime cheeks, to serve

JERK SEASONING

2 teaspoons sweet paprika
2 teaspoons garlic powder
1 teaspoon ground allspice
½ teaspoon cayenne pepper
¼ teaspoon ground nutmeg
½ teaspoon sea salt
¼ teaspoon freshly ground black pepper

ZESTY LIME CAULIFLOWER SMASH

1 head of cauliflower, broken into small florets
½ teaspoon smoked paprika
125 ml (½ cup) extra-virgin olive, avocado or macadamia oil, plus 2 tablespoons extra for drizzling
½ bunch of coriander, leaves picked
1 teaspoon garlic powder
finely grated zest and juice of 1 lime
sea salt and freshly ground black pepper

Preheat the oven to 180°C and line two baking trays with baking paper.

To make the jerk seasoning, mix all the ingredients in a bowl.

Add the oil, lemon zest and juice to the bowl with the jerk seasoning and mix well. Season with salt, then add the chicken drumsticks and toss well to coat. Leave to marinate for 15–30 minutes.

Meanwhile, make the cauliflower smash. Spread the cauliflower florets over one of the prepared baking trays. Sprinkle over the paprika, drizzle over 2 tablespoons of oil, then roast for 20–30 minutes, or until softened and lightly golden brown on the edges. Remove from the oven, transfer to a food processor and blitz with the oil, coriander, garlic powder and lime zest and juice to a rough but spreadable paste. Season to taste with salt and pepper and set aside.

When you're ready to cook the chicken, crank the oven up to 220°C and spread your drumsticks across the remaining baking tray in a single layer. Bake for 30–40 minutes, turning halfway through cooking, or until golden brown on the outside and cooked through.

Scatter the chopped coriander over the cauliflower smash and season well with salt and pepper. Serve with the drumsticks and lime cheeks for squeezing.

GOOD TO KNOW: *You can make the jerk seasoning in bulk if you like; simply multiply the batch and store the excess in an airtight container in the pantry for up to 3 months. I like adding it to pan-fried mince to pack it with flavour before serving it in crisp lettuce cups.*

HEALTH HACK: *Being a fattier cut of chicken, drumsticks are pretty nutrient dense. As a result, a little goes a long way and they will certainly keep you feeling fuller for longer than the lower-fat cuts, such as the breast.*

CHICKEN MOLE

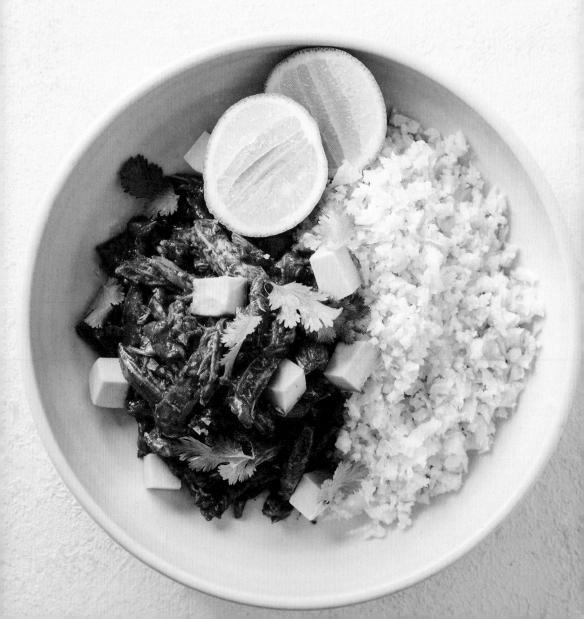

MOLE IS A TRADITIONAL MEXICAN SAUCE. PERHAPS BEST KNOWN FOR ITS USE OF CACAO IN A SAVOURY DISH, THIS SLIGHTLY SWEET AND SALTY SAUCE IS OFTEN PAIRED WITH BRAISED MEAT. IT'S SO RICH AND DELICIOUS, AND DOESN'T TASTE LIKE CHOCOLATE AT ALL. IT JUST TASTES YUM.

SERVES 4

800 g chicken thighs
sea salt and freshly ground
    black pepper
2 tablespoons coconut oil, grass-fed
    butter or ghee
1 onion, roughly chopped
2 garlic cloves, roughly chopped
250 ml (1 cup) chicken stock
    or bone broth
400 ml can coconut cream or
    coconut milk

MOLE SPICE MIX

3 tablespoons cacao powder
2 teaspoons ground cinnamon
1 teaspoon dried oregano
1 teaspoon chilli powder
½ teaspoon ground cumin
½ teaspoon ground coriander
½ teaspoon sea salt

TO SERVE

800 g (4 cups) Cauliflower Rice
    (see page 107)
1 avocado, halved and cut into cubes
1 handful of coriander leaves,
    roughly torn
1 lime, cut into cheeks

To make the mole spice mix, combine all the ingredients in a small bowl. Set aside.

Season the chicken thighs well with salt and pepper.

Heat your preferred cooking fat in a large frying pan over medium–high heat. Add the chicken and cook for 2–3 minutes on each side until lightly browned. Transfer to a plate and set aside.

Add the onion and garlic to the pan, reduce the heat to medium and saute for 4–5 minutes until softened and caramelised. Add the spice mix and cook, stirring, for 30 seconds until fragrant, then pour over the stock or broth. Deglaze the pan, using a wooden spoon to scrape any bits that are stuck to the bottom, then add the coconut cream or milk and bring to the boil.

Return the chicken and any juices to the pan, reduce the heat to low and simmer, turning the chicken occasionally, for 20–25 minutes, or until the sauce has reduced and thickened nicely.

Keeping the sauce warm over very low heat, remove the chicken pieces from the pan and set aside to cool slightly, then shred with a fork.

When ready to serve, return the shredded chicken to the pan, bring to a simmer and cook, stirring, for 5 minutes to heat through. Season with salt and pepper. Divide the mole and cauliflower rice among plates. Top with the avocado and coriander and serve with lime cheeks for squeezing.

GOOD TO KNOW: *To transform the mole into a thick, smooth sauce, once you've removed the chicken from the pan to shred it, blitz what's left with a stick blender to bring everything together. (This is totally optional, but it is super yum!)*

HEALTH HACK: *Raw cacao is rich in a number of minerals — and is particularly high in magnesium — making this recipe an excellent way of getting all this goodness into your system compared to the usual option of dark chocolate.*

ME

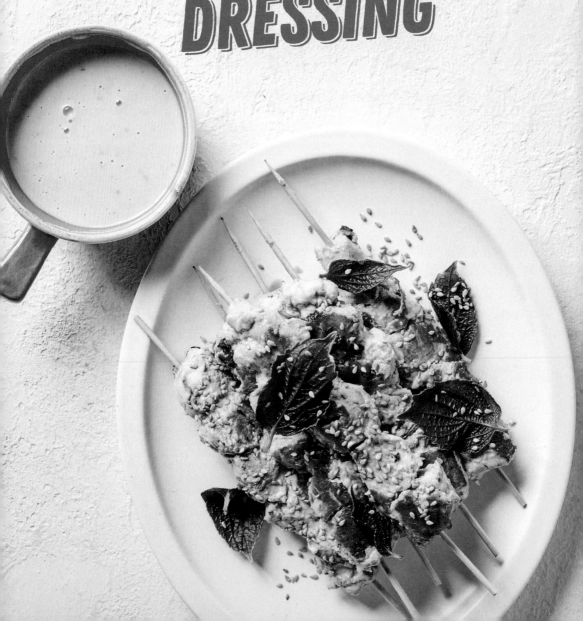

CHARGRILLED PORK SKEWERS with TAHINI DRESSING

TALK ABOUT SIMPLE AND DELICIOUS — THIS RECIPE IS A WONDERFUL WAY OF GETTING SOME MORE PORK ON YOUR FORK! THE TAHINI DRESSING IS SO EASY TO MAKE AND ACTS NOT ONLY AS A GREAT CONDIMENT ON TOP BUT ALSO AS A DELICIOUS MARINADE.

SERVES 4

800 g boneless pork tenderloin fillet,
    cut into 3 cm chunks
sesame seeds, toasted, to serve
1 red bird's eye chilli, finely
    sliced (optional)
1 small handful of shiso leaves
    (optional)
2 tablespoons extra-virgin olive oil

TAHINI DRESSING

135 g (½ cup) hulled tahini
125 ml (½ cup) canned coconut milk
2 tablespoons sugar-free fish sauce
1 tablespoon monk fruit syrup, maple
    syrup or raw honey
finely grated zest and juice of 2 limes
1 tablespoon extra-virgin olive,
    macadamia or avocado oil

Place eight large or twelve small bamboo skewers in a shallow dish, cover with cold water and leave to soak for at least 30 minutes.

To make the dressing, place all the ingredients in a bowl and whisk well.

Transfer half the dressing to a large bowl, add the pork pieces and turn to coat all over. Set aside to marinate for 15 minutes.

Preheat a chargrill pan or barbecue to medium.

Thread the marinated pork pieces onto the prepared skewers. Grill for 2–3 minutes on each side, or until cooked through and nicely charred and golden brown on the outside.

Transfer the skewers to a serving platter and scatter over the sesame seeds, chilli and shiso leaves (if using). Drizzle over the olive oil and serve with the remaining tahini dressing.

GOOD TO KNOW: *Pork tenderloin is a long, thinnish strip of lean meat. If you can't find any, simply pick up some pork loin – which is thicker and chunkier – and prepare it in the same way.*

HEALTH HACK: *Unlike other red meats such as beef and lamb, pork is particularly rich in thiamine – one of the B vitamins that is essential for good health.*

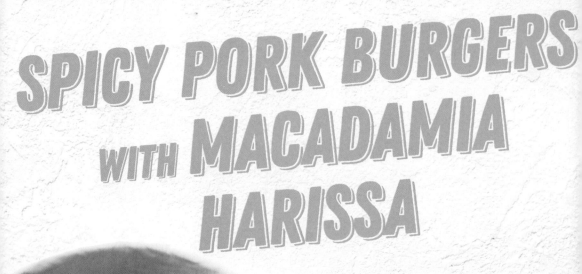

SPICY PORK BURGERS
WITH MACADAMIA
HARISSA

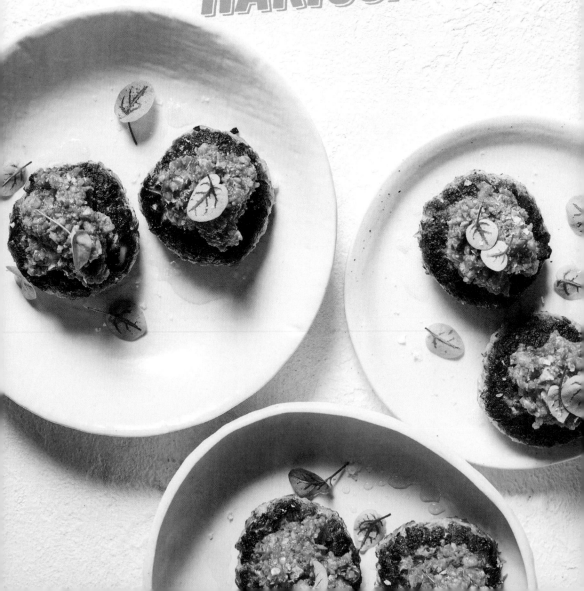

I LOVE RECIPES THAT ALLOW YOU TO COOK ONE COMPONENT WHILE PREPARING THE OTHER. HERE YOU CAN WHIP UP YOUR MACADAMIA HARISSA WHILE THE BURGERS ARE FIRING AWAY, AND DINNER WILL BE ON THE TABLE IN NO TIME AT ALL.

SERVES 4

3 tablespoons coconut oil, grass-fed butter or ghee
1 onion, finely diced
2 garlic cloves, very finely chopped
1 long red chilli, finely diced
600 g pork mince
2 tablespoons finely chopped flat-leaf parsley leaves
1 teaspoon dried chilli flakes
finely grated zest and juice of 1 lemon
sea salt and freshly ground black pepper
2 handfuls of salad leaves, such as sorrel, baby rocket or baby spinach (optional)

MACADAMIA HARISSA

3 tablespoons tomato paste
2 long red chillies, roughly chopped
3 tablespoons extra-virgin olive, avocado, macadamia or hemp oil
2 garlic cloves, crushed
½ teaspoon sea salt
1 teaspoon cumin seeds or ground cumin
1 teaspoon coriander seeds or ground coriander
1 teaspoon sweet or smoked paprika
finely grated zest and juice of 1 lemon
1 handful of coriander leaves
160 g (1 cup) macadamia nuts

Heat 1 tablespoon of your preferred cooking fat in a large frying pan over medium heat. Add the onion, garlic and chilli and cook, stirring, for 3–4 minutes until softened and caramelised. Remove from the heat and leave to cool slightly, then transfer to a large bowl and add the mince, parsley, chilli flakes and lemon zest and juice. Season with salt and pepper. Mix well with your hands, then shape into eight patties.

Heat the remaining cooking fat in the pan over medium heat, add the patties (in batches if necessary) and cook for 3–4 minutes on each side, or until cooked through and golden brown on the outside.

While your burgers are cooking, make the macadamia harissa. Blitz all the ingredients apart from the macadamias in a food processor until smooth. Add the macadamias and pulse briefly to form a thick, chunky paste.

Divide the burgers among plates, top with the macadamia harissa and scatter over the salad leaves, if desired.

GOOD TO KNOW: *This harissa is also great as a dip or condiment to serve with other proteins, such as fish or chicken, so make a large batch so that you have extra on hand (leftovers will keep in an airtight container in the fridge for up to 7 days). If you prefer a smoother finish, simply keep blitzing once you've added the macadamias to the processor.*

HEALTH HACK: *When going low carb, we are looking to replace the energy we receive from carbs with energy from good-quality fats, as these help us stay fuller for longer and energised all day long. So it's a case of the fattier the pork mince, the better here.*

SIMPLE STEAK WITH CHUNKY ROAST MASH

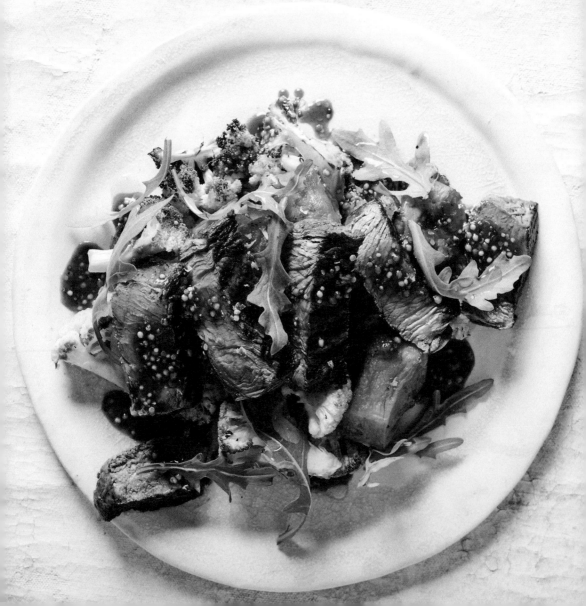

SOMETIMES SIMPLICITY IS KEY, ESPECIALLY WHEN IT COMES TO SENSATIONAL FLAVOURS. AND WHAT COULD BE MORE SENSATIONAL THAN A DELICIOUS STEAK AND VEG?

SERVES 4

4 x 150 g rump steaks, trimmed
sea salt and freshly ground
  black pepper
500 g cauliflower, broken into
  small florets
500 g butternut pumpkin, peeled and
  chopped into 2 cm chunks
3 tablespoons grass-fed butter
  or ghee
1 tablespoon wholegrain mustard
250 ml (1 cup) beef stock or
  bone broth
1 long red chilli, finely chopped
1 large handful of baby rocket leaves

Preheat the oven to 200°C and line two baking trays with baking paper.

Season the steaks with salt and pepper on both sides. Set aside.

Spread the cauliflower and pumpkin across the prepared trays, dot with 1 tablespoon of the butter or ghee and bake for 15–20 minutes, or until the pumpkin is soft enough to press with a fork and the cauliflower is golden brown.

Meanwhile, heat a large frying pan over medium–high heat. Working in two batches, add the steaks and cook for 2–3 minutes on each side for medium–rare, or until done to your liking. Transfer the cooked steaks to a plate and cover loosely with foil to rest. Return the pan to the heat, add the mustard and stock or broth and simmer for 2–3 minutes, or until the liquid is reduced by about half. Keep warm.

Transfer the roast veg to a bowl together with the chilli and remaining butter or ghee. Using the back of a fork, mix well to form a rough, chunky mash.

To serve, divide the mash among plates. Cut the steaks into thick slices and lay them over the mash. Spoon over the sauce and top with the baby rocket leaves to finish.

GOOD TO KNOW: *The rump is a slightly fattier cut of beef than other steaks, meaning it's packed with heaps of flavour. If you can't find a good rump steak, simply swap it out for another cut that you can find at your local butcher (preferably grass fed and organic).*

HEALTH HACK: *Using bone broth to make this lovely sauce not only gives it a delicious flavour, but also provides you with all the wonderful gut-healing benefits from the collagen and gelatine it contains. Pretty good going, huh?*

MEXICAN MEATBALLS
with SALSA SAUCE

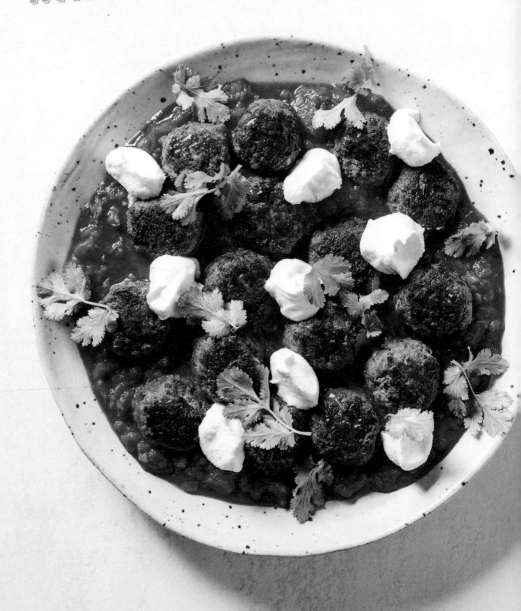

WHO DOESN'T LOVE A MEATBALL? HERE, I'VE TAKEN A SIMPLE TOMATO SALSA AND TRANSFORMED IT INTO A SENSATIONAL SPICY SAUCE TO GIVE THESE CLASSIC MEXICAN FLAVOURS A DELICIOUSLY DIFFERENT TAKE.

SERVES 4

600 g beef mince
1 bunch of coriander, leaves
    finely chopped
80 ml (⅓ cup) coconut oil, grass-fed
    butter or ghee, melted
1 egg
2 garlic cloves, very finely chopped
1 teaspoon ground cumin
1 teaspoon ground coriander
1 teaspoon dried chilli flakes
sea salt and freshly ground
    black pepper

MACADAMIA SOUR CREAM

160 g (1 cup) macadamia nuts, soaked
    in hot water for at least 15 minutes
juice of 1 lemon
2 teaspoons apple cider vinegar
½ teaspoon sea salt
80 ml (⅓ cup) filtered water

SALSA SAUCE

2 tablespoons coconut oil, grass-fed
    butter or ghee
1 onion, finely diced
2 garlic cloves, finely diced
2 long red chillies, finely diced
2 tomatoes, roughly diced
1 tablespoon tomato paste
1 teaspoon smoked paprika
1 teaspoon ground cumin
250 ml (1 cup) beef stock or
    bone broth
250 ml (1 cup) tomato passata

For the macadamia sour cream, drain the soaked nuts and rinse them really well, then transfer to a high-speed blender or food processor together with all the remaining ingredients and blitz for 1–2 minutes, or until beautifully smooth. Set aside.

Place the mince, half the coriander, 2 tablespoons of your preferred cooking fat, egg, garlic, spices, salt and pepper in a large bowl. Using your hands, mix everything really well. Roll the mixture into walnut-sized balls, transfer to a tray and place in the fridge for 30 minutes to firm.

While the meatballs are chilling, make the salsa sauce. Melt your preferred cooking fat in a large saucepan over medium heat. Add the onion, garlic and chilli, and saute for 4–5 minutes until softened and caramelised. Add the tomato, tomato paste and spices and cook, stirring, for a further 2 minutes. Stir in the stock or broth and tomato passata and bring to the boil, then reduce the heat and simmer for 15–20 minutes until thickened and reduced slightly.

Heat the remaining 2 tablespoons of your preferred cooking fat in a large frying pan over medium–high heat. Working in batches if necessary, add the meatballs to the pan and cook for 5–6 minutes until golden brown on all sides. Pour over the salsa sauce, bring to a simmer and cook for a further 8 minutes, or until the sauce is lovely and thick and the meatballs are cooked through.

Divide the meatballs among plates, scatter over the reserved coriander and season well with salt and pepper. Serve with generous dollops of the macadamia sour cream.

GOOD TO KNOW: *These meatballs are a great recipe to make in bulk. Whether cooked off first or transferred to an airtight container straight after shaping, they will keep in the fridge for up to 5 days and the freezer for up to 3 months.*

HEALTH HACK: *Looking to up your vegetable intake? Try adding some extra finely diced vegetables to the salsa sauce. Both mushroom and capsicum work well.*

KADDO BOURANI

SERVES 4

1 tablespoon coconut oil, grass-fed
   butter or ghee
1 onion, roughly diced
2 garlic cloves, roughly chopped
800 g beef mince (the fattier
   the better)
1 teaspoon ground turmeric
1 teaspoon ground coriander
½ teaspoon ground ginger
¼ teaspoon ground cinnamon
½ teaspoon dried chilli flakes
sea salt and freshly ground
   black pepper
250 ml (1 cup) beef stock, bone broth
   or filtered water
3 tablespoons tomato passata
1 handful of mint leaves

CREAMY YOGHURT SAUCE
125 ml (½ cup) canned
   coconut cream
125 g (½ cup) coconut yoghurt
finely grated zest and juice of
   1 lemon
1 garlic clove, very finely chopped
½ bunch of mint, leaves
   finely chopped

PUMPKIN
1 kg kent pumpkin, unpeeled,
   deseeded and cut into 4 wedges
1 tablespoon extra-virgin olive oil
1 teaspoon ground cumin
1 teaspoon ground coriander
sea salt and freshly ground
   black pepper

Preheat the oven to 180°C and line a large baking tray with baking paper.

To make the creamy yoghurt sauce, mix all the ingredients in a small bowl. Set aside in the fridge to chill.

For the pumpkin, place the pumpkin wedges on the prepared tray, drizzle over the olive oil and sprinkle over the spices. Using your hands, massage the pumpkin pieces so they are well coated in the spiced oil. Season generously with salt and pepper and roast for 45 minutes, or until the pumpkin is golden brown and soft.

Meanwhile, melt your preferred cooking fat in a large frying pan over medium heat. Add the onion and garlic and saute for 2–3 minutes until softened and caramelised, then add the mince and cook for 5–6 minutes, breaking any lumps with a wooden spoon as you cook, until browned all over. Add the spices and season generously with salt, then stir through the stock, broth or water and tomato paste. Bring to the boil, then reduce the heat and simmer, uncovered, for 10–15 minutes, or until the liquid has mostly evaporated.

To serve, divide the pumpkin wedges among shallow bowls, spoon over the mince and top with the yoghurt sauce. Scatter over the mint leaves, season well with salt and pepper and enjoy.

GOOD TO KNOW: *Afghan food is very well known for incorporating yoghurt into savoury dishes like this, but if you fancy mixing things up a bit, you could always try replacing it with the macadamia sour cream on page 145 instead.*

HEALTH HACK: *I always use full-fat coconut cream or unsweetened coconut yoghurt as my preferred non-dairy alternative. When things are labelled as reduced fat, sometimes they add sugar to make them taste good — one of many reasons we should always stick with the real deal. Here's to keeping it as natural as possible, legends!*

BOTH COMFORTING AND MOREISH, THIS AFGHANI FAVOURITE IS ALL ABOUT THE KILLER COMBO OF MELT-IN-THE-MOUTH ROAST PUMPKIN, FLAVOURSOME MINCE AND SAVOURY YOGHURT. TRY IT ONCE AND YOU'LL FIND ANY EXCUSE TO HAVE IT AGAIN.

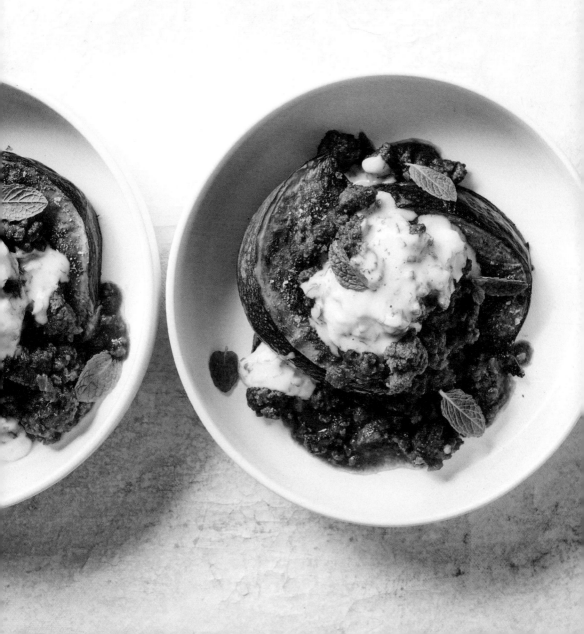

MINUTE STEAK AND BUTTERY MUSHROOMS

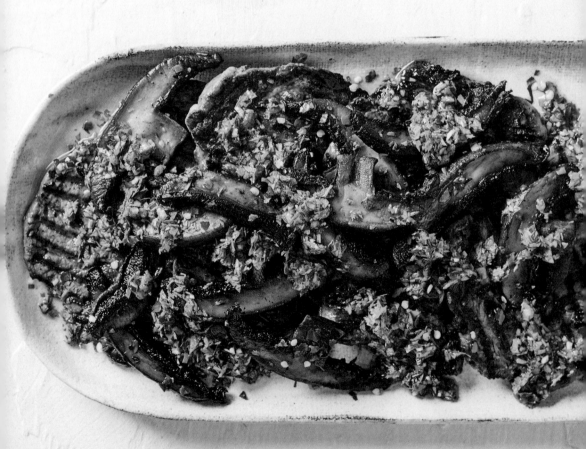

THE GARLICKY MUSHROOMS AND CHIMICHURRI REALLY DO MAKE FOR THE PERFECT FLAVOUR COMBO IN THIS SIMPLE RECIPE THAT'S PERFECT FOR ANY NIGHT OF THE WEEK.

SERVES 4

3 tablespoons grass-fed butter, melted
400 g portobello mushrooms, cut into
    4 cm thick strips
2 garlic cloves, finely chopped
sea salt and freshly ground
    black pepper
8 x 80 g minute steaks
2 teaspoons dried chilli flakes
125 ml (½ cup) Chimichurri
    (see page 80)

Heat half the butter in a large frying pan over medium heat. Add the mushrooms and saute for 3–4 minutes until softened and tender, then add the garlic and continue to cook for 1–2 minutes until lightly golden brown. Season well with salt and keep warm over very low heat.

Heat a chargrill pan or barbecue grill to high.

Brush the steaks with the remaining butter and season well with salt and pepper. Cook for 1–2 minutes on each side, or until cooked to your liking.

Pile the steaks and mushrooms onto a large platter and top with the dried chilli flakes and dollops of chimichurri.

GOOD TO KNOW: *Minute steaks are super thin, which is why they don't take long to cook. The key is to cook them over a very high heat and to keep a close eye on them – you want the steaks to still be a bit pink in the middle.*

HEALTH HACK: *Mushrooms contain such an amazing range of healthy bacteria that they almost deserve to be counted as their own food group. Indeed, some of these bacteria strains cannot be found in anything else we eat, making them an essential component to good gut health.*

BANGIN' BURGERS with MUSHROOM BUNS

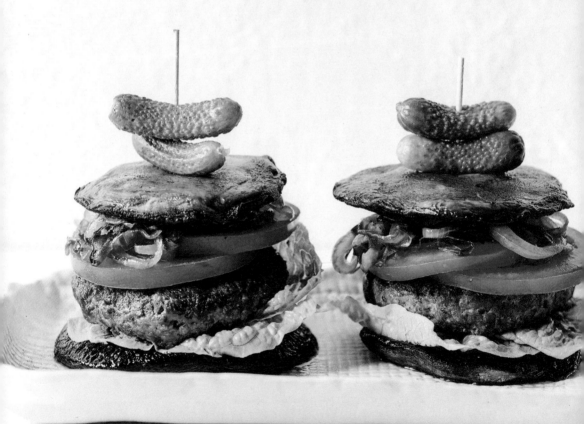

IT'S A WELL-KNOWN FACT THAT I LOVE A JUICY BURGER. YUM. BUT WHAT I LOVE MOST OF ALL IS A BURGER THAT I CAN WHIP UP EASILY WITHOUT THE NEED FOR BREAD OR BUNS. WITH ITS CLEVER MUSHROOM BUNS AND FLAVOUR-PACKED CARAMELISED ONIONS, THIS ONE'S A WINNER ON ALL COUNTS.

MAKES 4

400 g beef mince
1 egg
2 tablespoons finely chopped flat-leaf
   parsley leaves
2 teaspoons dried rosemary
1 teaspoon dried chilli flakes
sea salt and freshly ground
   black pepper
2 tablespoons coconut oil, grass-fed
   butter or ghee, plus extra if needed
1 red onion, sliced into rings
8 large portobello mushrooms
1 baby gem lettuce, leaves separated
1 tomato, finely sliced
8 small unsweetened gherkins

Place the mince, egg, parsley, rosemary and chilli in a large bowl. Season with salt and pepper and, using your hands, mix everything really well. Shape into four equal-sized balls, then gently flatten them to form 3 cm thick patties. Place on a tray and transfer to the fridge for 10 minutes to firm up.

Remove the patties from the fridge and leave for about 10 minutes to come back to room temperature.

Melt your preferred cooking fat in a large frying pan over medium–high heat. Add the patties and cook for 2–3 minutes each side, or until golden brown and cooked through. Transfer to a plate, cover loosely with foil and set aside to rest.

Add a little more cooking fat to the pan if needed, along with half the onion and mushrooms, stem-side down. Cook for 4–6 minutes, turning the mushrooms halfway through cooking, or until the onion has softened and caramelised and the mushrooms are soft and tender. Transfer to a plate and repeat with the remaining onion and mushrooms.

To plate up, start with a mushroom, stem-side up, on the plate, then layer over a few lettuce leaves followed by one of the burger patties, some tomato and caramelised onion. Top the whole thing with another mushroom, stem-side down, then use a toothpick to add some gherkins on top. Repeat with the rest of the ingredients and dig in!

GOOD TO KNOW: *I don't mind these burgers being a bit of a handful, but you can always hold them together with a wooden skewer if you like. They are particularly good paired with the Baked Butternut Fries on page 86.*

HEALTH HACK: *Given that the average burger bun contains more than 30 g of carbs per serve, using mushrooms instead can make a dramatic difference to your daily carb intake.*

SRI LANKAN LAMB ROAST AND REALLY GOOD RAITA

SERVES 4

3 tablespoons extra-virgin olive oil, grass-fed butter or ghee, melted
1.5 kg bone-in lamb shoulder
5 garlic cloves, very finely chopped
1 teaspoon garam masala
½ teaspoon ground cumin
½ teaspoon ground coriander
1 teaspoon ground cardamom
sea salt and freshly ground black pepper
250 ml (1 cup) beef stock, chicken stock or filtered water
125 ml (½ cup) canned coconut milk or cream
1 kg butternut pumpkin, cut into 6 cm chunks
3 tablespoons shredded coconut, toasted
1 handful of coriander leaves

RAITA

125 g (½ cup) coconut yoghurt
2 Lebanese cucumbers, cut into 2 cm chunks
½ bunch of mint, leaves roughly chopped
finely grated zest and juice of 1 lemon
sea salt and freshly ground black pepper

Preheat the oven to 160°C and grease a large baking dish with 1 tablespoon of your preferred cooking fat.

To make the raita, mix all the ingredients in a bowl. Set aside in the fridge until ready to serve.

Place the lamb in the prepared baking dish and top with the garlic, spices and a generous seasoning of salt. Drizzle over the remaining 2 tablespoons of your preferred cooking fat and use your hands to massage all the flavourings into the lamb, getting good coverage all over.

Pour the stock or water and coconut milk or cream into the dish, cover with foil and roast for 3 hours. Remove the foil and roast for a further 3 hours, scattering the pumpkin over the base of the dish for the final 45 minutes, or until the pumpkin is golden brown and the meat is tender and falling apart at the touch of a fork.

Remove the dish from the oven and transfer to the centre of the table. Season well with salt and pepper, scatter over the coconut and coriander and serve straight from the dish with the raita on the side.

GOOD TO KNOW: *This goes really wonderfully with the garlic flatbreads on page 80. Just pile some shredded lettuce over one of the breads, top it with some of the lamb and a dollop or two of raita and wrap it up for an amazing lamb souvlaki.*

HEALTH HACK: *Lamb is a particularly fantastic source of vitamin B12, which aids in energy and brain function.*

SRI LANKAN CUISINE MAKES GREAT USE OF A DIVERSE RANGE OF HERBS AND SPICES TO CREATE FOOD THAT IS FLAVOURSOME, RICH AND VIBRANT. THIS LAMB SHOULDER IS PERFECT FOR BOTH SHARING AT A DINNER WITH FRIENDS, OR ENJOYING SOLO WITH LOTS OF LOVELY LEFTOVERS FOR THE WEEK AHEAD.

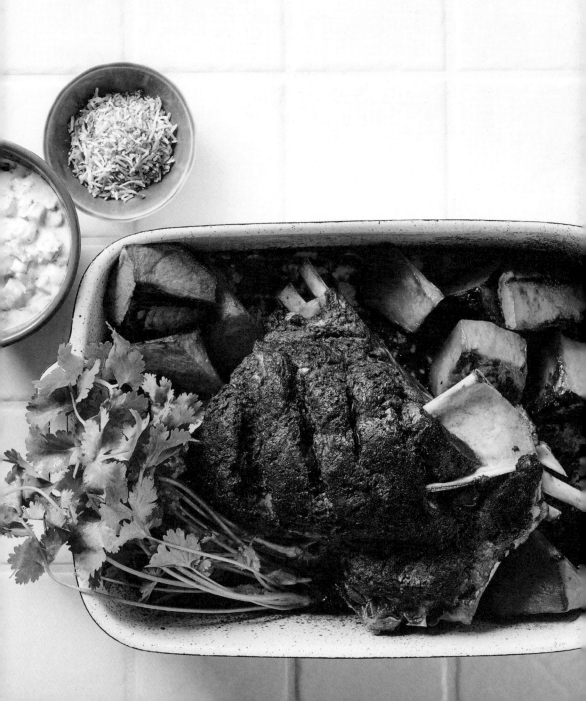

MARINATED LAMB KOFTA WITH TERRIFIC TURMERIC SAUCE

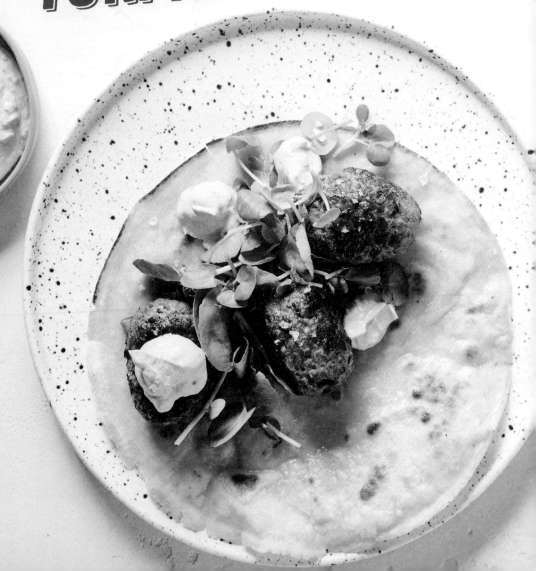

KOFTA IS A GENERAL TERM FOR THE SPICED MEATBALLS THAT ARE COMMON IN MEDITERRANEAN, MIDDLE EASTERN AND INDIAN COOKING. ALTHOUGH THEY ARE OFTEN COOKED ON SKEWERS, HERE WE ROLL THEM INTO OVALS INSTEAD, THOUGH YOU CAN ALWAYS SHAPE THEM INTO MEATBALLS OR EVEN PATTIES IF YOU WISH. THE SKY'S THE LIMIT!

SERVES 4

500 g lamb mince
1 teaspoon sea salt
1 teaspoon garlic powder
1 teaspoon chopped fresh or
   dried rosemary
1 tablespoon finely chopped
   mint leaves
½ bunch of flat-leaf parsley, leaves
   finely chopped
½ onion, finely chopped
watercress or rocket, to serve

TERRIFIC TURMERIC SAUCE

2 tablespoons macadamia or
   peanut butter
2 tablespoons extra-virgin olive,
   avocado or macadamia oil
2 tablespoons apple cider vinegar
2 garlic cloves, very finely chopped
1 tablespoon hulled tahini
½ teaspoon ground turmeric
finely grated zest and juice of 1 lemon
sea salt and freshly ground
   black pepper
1–2 tablespoons filtered
   water (optional)

FLATBREADS

100 g (1 cup) almond meal
125 g (1 cup) arrowroot or
   tapioca flour
125 ml (½ cup) canned coconut milk
2 eggs
125 ml (½ cup) filtered water
sea salt
2–3 tablespoons coconut oil

Place the mince, salt, garlic powder, herbs and onion in a large bowl. Using your hands, mix everything really well. Divide the mixture into eight portions and form each into an oval shape. Refrigerate for 20 minutes.

For the sauce, place all the ingredients in a food processor or high-speed blender and pulse until combined. Add a tablespoon or two of warm water to achieve your desired consistency if necessary, then set aside in the fridge ready for serving.

For the flatbreads, combine the almond meal, arrowroot or tapioca flour, coconut milk, eggs and water in a bowl. Mix well and season with salt. Melt 1 tablespoon of coconut oil in a small non-stick frying pan over medium heat. Ladle a quarter of the batter into the pan, tilting and swirling it to coat the base in an even layer, and cook for 2–3 minutes. Carefully turn the flatbread over with a spatula and cook for a further 2 minutes, or until golden and cooked through. Lift the flatbread from the pan and set aside, wrapped in a clean tea towel to keep warm. Repeat with the remaining mixture, greasing the pan with a little more coconut oil in between flatbreads to make sure they don't stick to the pan.

Remove the kofta from the fridge and leave for 5–10 minutes to come back to room temperature.

Heat a chargrill pan or barbecue grill to medium–high.

Cook the kofta for 3–4 minutes on each side, or until golden brown and caramelised on the outside and cooked through but still a little pink.

To serve, divide the flatbreads among plates and top with the koftas. Add a handful of watercress or rocket, spoon over the turmeric sauce, wrap up and devour.

HEALTH HACK: *Often touted as the anti-inflammatory spice, turmeric requires both good-quality fat and freshly ground black pepper to be absorbed well by our body. So don't hold back on either to make the most of this delicious sauce.*

TRE

ATS

LUKE'S BLOCK OF CHOC

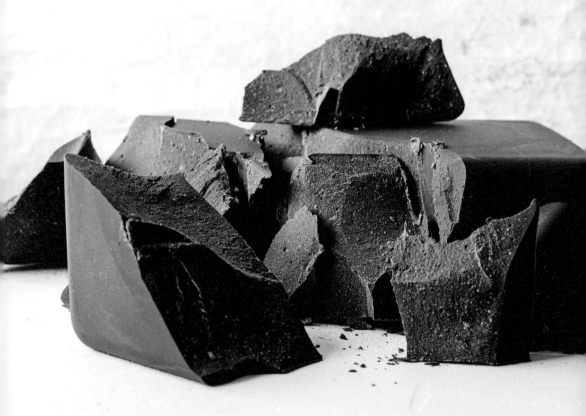

THIS IS POSSIBLY MY FAVOURITE VERSION OF MY HOMEMADE LOW-CARB CHOCOLATE. TO KEEP THINGS SIMPLE, I'VE STRIPPED IT BACK TO BASICS SO YOU CAN EITHER MAKE A BIG BATCH OF CHOC AND USE IT IN THE RECIPES THROUGHOUT THIS BOOK, OR FLAVOUR IT WITH THE IDEAS IN THE TIP BELOW.

MAKES ABOUT 400 G

220 g cacao butter

250 ml (1 cup) coconut oil, plus
  extra if needed

250 g (2 cups) cacao powder,
  plus extra if needed

1 teaspoon vanilla bean paste
  or powder

2–4 drops of liquid stevia or
  250 ml (1 cup) monk fruit syrup,
  plus extra if needed

Line a baking tray or loaf tin with baking paper.

In a saucepan over medium–low heat, gently stir the cacao butter and coconut oil until melted and well combined.

Remove the pan from the heat and gently whisk in the cacao power, vanilla and your sweetener of choice. Keep whisking until thick, creamy and well combined, then taste and evaluate the consistency and sweetness as follows:

For a thicker, darker chocolate, add some more cacao powder.

For a smoother chocolate, add some more coconut oil.

For a sweeter chocolate, add some more sweetener of choice.

Once the chocolate has reached your desired taste and consistency, pour it into the prepared tray or tin, transfer to the fridge or freezer and leave until set firm. Store in an airtight container in the fridge for up to 1 month, or in the freezer for up to 3 months.

GOOD TO KNOW: *This chocolate can easily be flavoured with your favourite ingredients. To do so, simply pour the chocolate into the tray as above and then sprinkle over your chosen nuts, seeds and fresh or freeze-dried berries. You can also swirl in soft ingredients like peanut butter or tahini, then set as above. Delicious.*

HEALTH HACK: *You'll see that any recipe that calls for chocolate in this book uses this chocolate. The reason for this is that, not only is it really good for you, it's also a great recipe to make in bulk and have on hand for when you want to get creative. But if you really don't have time to make it, you can always swap it out for a good-quality dark chocolate with 90% cocoa solids.*

LOW-CARB LAMINGTONS

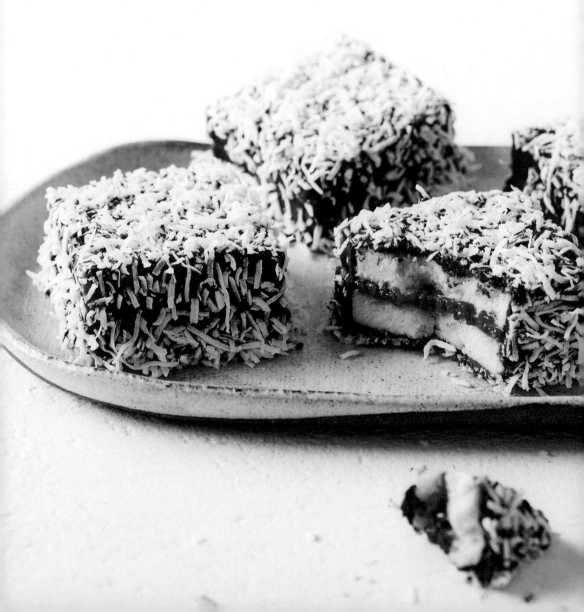

I ABSOLUTELY LOVE LAMINGTONS AND THIS LOWER-CARB VERSION REALLY HITS THE SPOT. WHETHER YOU GIVE THESE A GO FOR AUSTRALIA DAY OR GET CRACKING ON THEM RIGHT NOW, YOU'LL FIND THIS IS ONE KILLER RECIPE.

MAKES 6

VANILLA SPONGE

200 g (2 cups) almond meal
1 teaspoon gluten-free baking powder
1 teaspoon vanilla bean powder
   or extract
125 ml (½ cup) monk fruit syrup,
   coconut nectar or maple syrup
125 ml (½ cup) canned coconut
   cream
3 eggs
pinch of sea salt
80 ml (⅓ cup) filtered water
100 g unsalted grass-fed butter or
   ghee, melted

RASPBERRY JAM

250 g (2 cups) frozen raspberries
2 tablespoons white chia seeds
2 tablespoons filtered water

CHOCOLATE COATING

400 g Luke's Block of Choc
   (see page 158), melted and cooled
   to room temperature
90 g (1 cup) desiccated coconut

Preheat the oven to 180°C and line a 20 cm square cake tin with baking paper.

To make the vanilla sponge, place the almond meal, baking powder, vanilla and sweetener of choice in a bowl and mix well. Add the coconut cream, eggs, salt, water and melted butter or ghee and stir to form a batter. Pour the mixture into the prepared cake tin and bake for 35–40 minutes, or until lightly golden on top and a skewer inserted into the centre comes out clean. Remove from the oven and leave to cool completely.

While the cake is cooling, make the raspberry jam. Place all the ingredients in a saucepan over medium–high heat, cover with a lid and bring to the boil. Reduce the heat and simmer, uncovered, for 15–20 minutes until reduced and slightly thickened. Remove from the heat and leave to cool and thicken further.

Slice the cake into six even squares, then cut each square in half horizontally. Spread a small amount of the raspberry jam over the cut side of the bottom pieces, then sandwich with the top pieces. Transfer to a wire rack, then place the rack in the fridge to chill for 15–20 minutes.

For the chocolate coating, place the chocolate in a bowl. Place the desiccated coconut in another bowl.

Remove the rack from the fridge and set it on top of a baking tray. Spoon the cooled melted chocolate evenly over the chilled lamingtons and sprinkle over the desiccated coconut, then return to the fridge for 10–15 minutes for the chocolate to set. Enjoy!

GOOD TO KNOW: *Feel free to mix this recipe up by swapping the raspberries for blueberries.*

HEALTH HACK: *Chia seeds are not only rich in nutrients and omega-3 fats, they are also high in antioxidants and fibre. If you're a fan, try adding them to smoothies or have a go at whipping up my pudding on page 44.*

COCONUT CARROT CAKE

SERVES 8–10

200 g (2 cups) almond meal

60 g (1 cup) shredded coconut, toasted

120 g (1 cup) pecans, roughly chopped, toasted, plus 3 tablespoons extra to decorate

2 teaspoons gluten-free baking powder

1 teaspoon ground cloves

1 teaspoon ground cinnamon

1 teaspoon ground ginger

1 teaspoon vanilla bean paste or extract

6 eggs, beaten

200 g unsalted grass-fed butter, melted

4–6 drops of liquid stevia or 125 ml (½ cup) monk fruit syrup

3 carrots (about 300 g), grated

edible flowers, to decorate (optional)

LEMON BUTTER FROSTING

250 g coconut butter

125 ml (½ cup) coconut oil

2–4 drops of liquid stevia or 125 ml (½ cup) monk fruit syrup

finely grated zest and juice of 1 lemon

Preheat the oven to 180°C and line a 20 cm cake tin with baking paper.

In a large bowl, combine the almond meal, coconut, pecans, baking powder, spices and vanilla.

In a separate large bowl, whisk the egg, butter and sweetener of choice. Fold in the grated carrot.

Add the dry ingredients to the wet and stir well, then pour the mixture into the prepared tin and bake for 45 minutes, or until a skewer inserted into the centre comes out clean. Leave it to cool completely in the tin before carefully turning out onto a board or serving plate.

For the frosting, melt the coconut butter and coconut oil in a saucepan over low heat, add your sweetener of choice, lemon zest and juice, and stir to combine. Transfer to a bowl and place in the fridge for 10–15 minutes to thicken slightly. It should be spreadable and thick – be careful not to leave it for too long or it will set rock hard.

To serve, spread the frosting over the cake and decorate with the extra pecans and edible flowers, if using.

___

GOOD TO KNOW: *Instead of making this in a cake tin, you can use a 12-hole muffin tray if you like. Just reduce the baking time to 25–30 minutes, or until the cakes are golden brown and crunchy on top.*

HEALTH HACK: *While carrots may not help you see in the dark, the vitamin A does help to prevent vision loss.*

EVERY YEAR CARROT CAKE IS VOTED ONE OF THE WORLD'S TOP FIVE FAVOURITE CAKES. IT'S NOT HARD TO SEE WHY, ESPECIALLY IF YOU GIVE THIS HEALTHIER TAKE A TRY. HERE THE DELICIOUSNESS OF SHREDDED COCONUT HAS BEEN ADDED TO THOSE FAMILIAR SPICES, ALONG WITH A HIT OF COCONUT BUTTER IN THE FROSTING FOR GOOD MEASURE. YUM!

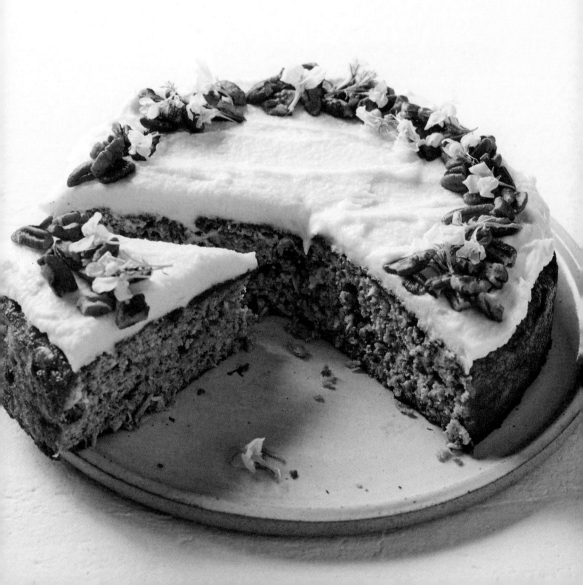

MUM'S MINT SLICE

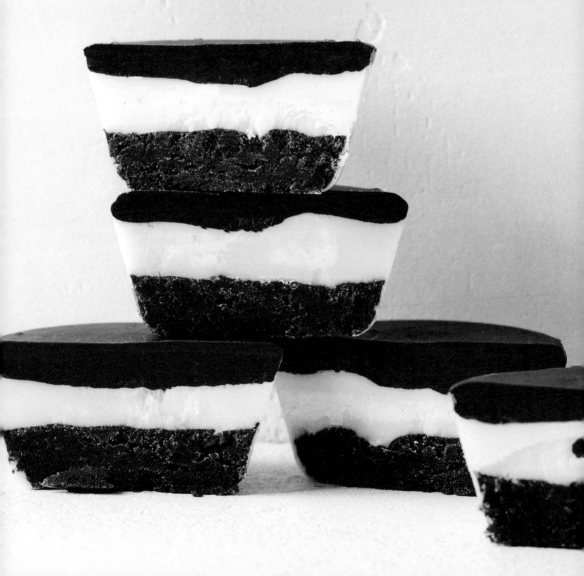

MY MUM AND I ARE MASSIVE FANS OF THE MINT SLICE BISCUIT, AND OVER THE YEARS I HAVE BEEN WORKSHOPPING AND TWEAKING THE ULTIMATE HEALTHY VERSION. I RECKON THIS ONE'S PRETTY AWESOME – TELL ME WHAT YOU THINK!

MAKES 12

BISCUIT BASE
125 g (½ cup) peanut or
    almond butter
1 egg
3 tablespoons monk fruit syrup,
    maple syrup or coconut nectar
2 tablespoons cacao powder
pinch of sea salt

MINT FILLING
125 ml (½ cup) coconut oil
200 g (1 cup) coconut butter
2–4 drops of peppermint essential oil
2–4 drops of liquid stevia or
    2 tablespoons monk fruit syrup

CHOCOLATE TOPPING
200 g Luke's Block of Choc (see page
    158), melted

Preheat the oven to 160°C and line a 12-hole muffin tray with silicone or paper cases.

For the biscuit base, mix all the ingredients in a bowl. Divide the mixture evenly among the muffin holes, then use your fingers to press it down to create an even, flat layer. Bake for 12–15 minutes, or until set and slightly coming away from the edges. Remove from the oven and leave to cool completely.

For the mint filling, melt the coconut oil and coconut butter in a saucepan over medium–low heat, stirring until well combined. Remove from the heat and stir in the peppermint oil and your sweetener of choice. Set aside to cool slightly, then spoon the mixture over the biscuit layer in the muffin tray, using about 1 tablespoon per hole. Transfer to the freezer for 30 minutes for the mint layer to set completely.

For the chocolate topping, melt the chocolate in a small saucepan over low heat, stirring, until thick and creamy. Remove from the heat and leave to cool slightly so that it is still runny but not super hot.

Once the mint filling is set, remove the tray from the freezer and pour the melted chocolate evenly over the top to cover completely. Return to the freezer for another 30 minutes or until the chocolate topping has set completely.

When ready to serve, remove the slices from the tray and leave to soften and come to room temperature. Enjoy.

GOOD TO KNOW: *These are best stored in the fridge for a soft, biteable filling, and will keep in an airtight container for up to 7 days. They can also be frozen for up to 3 months – just be sure to let them thaw before eating.*

HEALTH HACK: *As well as being a flavoursome addition to many different treat recipes, essential oils are also loaded with polyphenols that trigger a number of positive immune, hormonal and metabolism responses within your body.*

GREEN APPLE MUFFINS

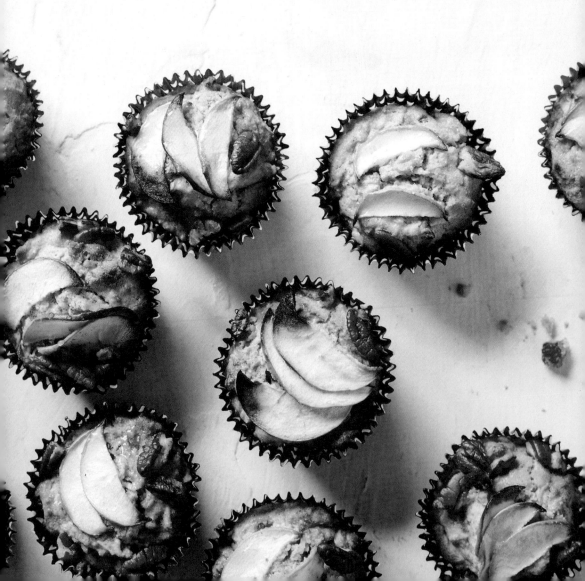

THESE MUFFINS ARE A FANTASTIC RECIPE TO MAKE AT THE START OF THE WEEK FOR WHEN YOU NEED A HEALTHY SNACK. THESE BEAUTIES WILL CURB CRAVINGS AS THE SWEETNESS COMES FROM GREEN APPLES, WHICH HAVE A LOWER FRUCTOSE CONTENT.

MAKES 12

200 g (2 cups) almond meal
100 g (1 cup) pecans, toasted
  and roughly chopped
60 g (1 cup) shredded coconut,
  lightly toasted
1 teaspoon gluten-free baking powder
1 teaspoon ground cinnamon
1 teaspoon vanilla bean powder
  or paste
4 eggs, beaten
125 ml (½ cup) coconut oil, melted
2 green apples, grated

TOPPING

2 tablespoons roughly chopped
  pecans, toasted
1 green apple, sliced into thin
  half-moons

Preheat the oven to 180°C and line a 12-hole muffin tray with paper cases.

Combine all the dry ingredients in a large bowl. Stirring as you go, slowly add the egg, coconut oil and apple to form a batter.

Spoon the batter into the prepared tray and top with the toasted pecans and apple slices. Bake for 30–40 minutes, or until the muffins are golden brown on top and a skewer inserted into the centre of one of them comes out clean. Remove from the oven and leave to cool before eating.

GOOD TO KNOW: *These can be stored in an airtight container in the fridge for up to 5 days or the freezer for up to 3 months. And feel free to experiment here – try adding a little grated carrot or a few low-fructose mixed berries for extra flavour and colour.*

HEALTH HACK: *Green apples have been shown to be chock-full of antioxidants that can help keep our skin elastic and fight off wrinkles. An apple a day? Don't mind if I do.*

WHITE CHOCOLATE 'ROCHERS'

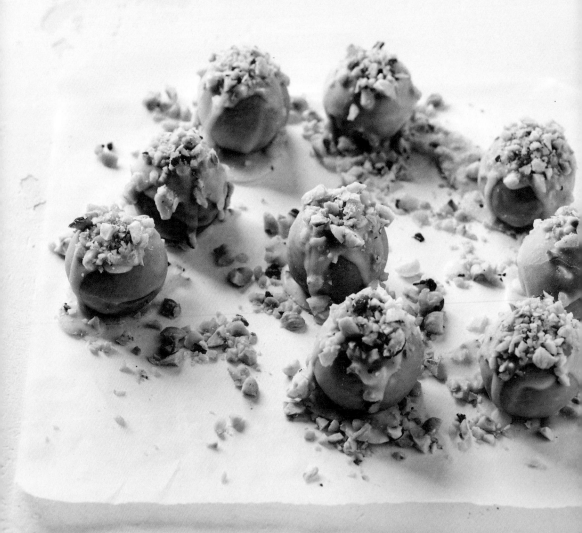

WHO DOESN'T LOVE A FERRERO ROCHER? HERE'S MY WHITE CHOCOLATE SPIN ON THIS CLASSIC FAVOURITE.

MAKES 12

'FERRERO' FILLING
250 g (1 cup) hazelnut butter
125 g (½ cup) coconut butter, melted
110 g (½ cup) raw cacao butter,
    melted
4–6 drops of liquid stevia or
    3 tablespoons monk fruit syrup,
    maple syrup or coconut nectar

WHITE CHOCOLATE COATING
110 g (½ cup) raw cacao
    butter, melted
125 g (½ cup) coconut butter
4–6 drops of liquid stevia or
    3 tablespoons monk fruit syrup,
    maple syrup or coconut nectar
1 teaspoon vanilla bean paste
    or extract
60 g (½ cup) roughly chopped
    toasted hazelnuts

For the filling, blitz all the ingredients in a food processor or high-speed blender to form a thick paste.

Spoon the filling mixture evenly into 24 half-sphere silicone chocolate moulds, each about 30 mm in diameter. Transfer to the freezer and leave for 1 hour to chill and firm.

Meanwhile, for the white chocolate coating, warm the cacao butter, coconut butter, sweetener of choice and vanilla in a saucepan over very low heat. Stir gently until well combined, then set aside to cool slightly.

Once chilled, unmould the half spheres. Press the flat side of each half sphere on a warm, flat surface to melt the filling slightly, then press another half sphere on top to join and form a complete sphere. Using a spoon, lower the sphere into the white chocolate to coat, then transfer to a wire rack set over a chopping board. Sprinkle with the chopped hazelnuts. Repeat with the remaining ingredients, then return to the freezer to set for 20–30 minutes. (If you'd like a thicker white chocolate coating, before sprinkling with the hazelnuts, re-freeze the spheres with one layer, then do another layer before applying the nuts.)

GOOD TO KNOW: *If you don't have any silicone moulds, you can make these by hand but it will take a little longer. Transfer your filling to the fridge and check on it every 15 minutes. Once it is a malleable paste, work quickly to roll it into 12 even balls with your hands, then transfer to the freezer to set and continue as above.*

HEALTH HACK: *Hazelnuts are a super-healthy nut. They have many health benefits including protecting against cell damage, lowering levels of cholesterol and improving insulin sensitivity.*

TEMPTING TRUFFLES WITH COLLAGEN

MAKES 15

200 g Luke's Block of Choc (see page 158)
2 tablespoons cacao nibs
2 tablespoons freeze-dried raspberries, crushed into small chunks

COLLAGEN FILLING

500 g (2 cups) hazelnut, macadamia or cashew butter
125 ml (½ cup) coconut oil, melted
60 g (½ cup) cacao powder
3 tablespoons cacao butter, melted
4–6 drops of stevia or 125 ml (½ cup) monk fruit syrup,
2 tablespoons plain collagen powder (see Health Hack)

For the collagen filling, blitz the ingredients in a food processor or high-speed blender until smooth. Spoon the mixture into 15 silicone moulds and place in the freezer to firm up for at least 1 hour.

Melt the chocolate in a small saucepan over low heat, stirring, until thick and creamy. Remove from the heat and leave to cool slightly so that it is still runny but not super hot.

When you're ready to bring the elements together, remove the silicone moulds from the freezer and take the fillings out of the moulds. Using a spoon, lower one into the melted chocolate to coat completely, then transfer to a wire rack set over a chopping board and sprinkle over the cacao nibs and raspberries. Repeat with the rest of the fillings, then place the truffles in the fridge until the chocolate is set and they are ready to be devoured.

<u>GOOD TO KNOW:</u> *If you don't have any silicone moulds, you can do these by hand — just follow the instructions in Good to Know on page 169. For a thicker chocolate coating, before sprinkling over with the cacao nibs and raspberries, re-freeze the truffles with one layer of chocolate until set, then repeat with a second layer before applying the toppings.*

<u>HEALTH HACK:</u> *Taking collagen has been associated with a number of health benefits. For starters, supplementing with powdered collagen in your diet may improve skin health by reducing wrinkles and skin dryness, in addition to potentially increasing lean muscle mass, preventing bone loss and relieving joint pain.*

COLLAGEN IS THE MOST ABUNDANT PROTEIN IN OUR BODIES. IT HAS MANY IMPORTANT FUNCTIONS, INCLUDING PROVIDING OUR SKIN WITH STRUCTURE AND STRENGTHENING OUR BONES. MOST OF THE POWDERS YOU'LL FIND IN-STORE AND ONLINE ARE HYDROLYSED, WHICH MEANS THE COLLAGEN HAS BEEN BROKEN DOWN, MAKING IT EASIER FOR US TO ABSORB. ADDING A LITTLE COLLAGEN TO THESE TRUFFLES REALLY INCREASES THEIR ALREADY IMPRESSIVE HEALTH BENEFITS.

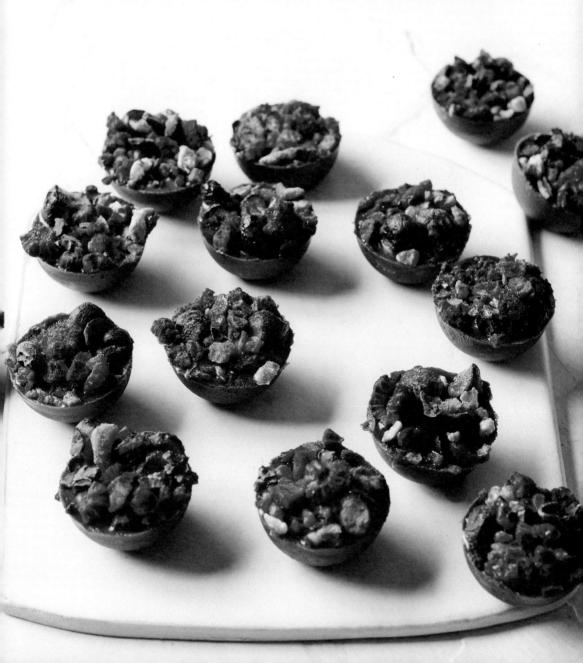

APPLE AND BERRY CRUMBLE CUPS

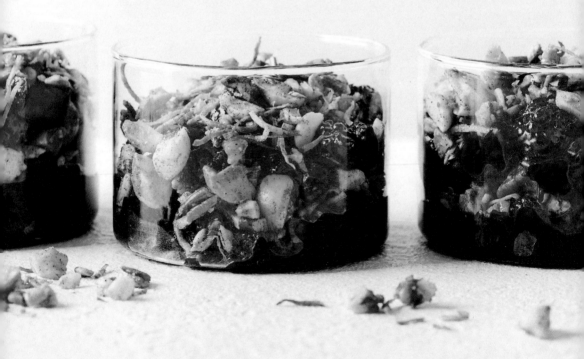

I LOVE A TRADITIONAL CRUMBLE BUT THESE LITTLE CUPS ARE A PARTICULARLY SPECIAL WAY TO SERVE THIS CLASSIC DESSERT. AND THEY CAN BE WHIPPED UP IN NO TIME, WHICH MAKES THEM THE PERFECT TREAT FOR ANY DAY OF THE WEEK.

SERVES 4

2 tablespoons coconut oil, grass-fed butter or ghee
2 green apples, cut into 1 cm chunks
500 g (4 cups) mixed berries (fresh or frozen)
2 tablespoons monk fruit syrup, maple syrup or coconut nectar (optional)

CRUMBLE

160 g (1 cup) macadamia nuts, roughly chopped
60 g (1 cup) shredded coconut
50 (½ cup) pecans, roughly chopped
60 (½ cup) pumpkin seeds
2 tablespoons monk fruit syrup, maple syrup or coconut nectar
2 tablespoons coconut oil, grass-fed butter or ghee
1 teaspoon ground cinnamon
1 teaspoon vanilla bean powder or extract

Preheat the oven to 160°C and line a large baking tray with baking paper.

For the crumble, mix all the ingredients in a large bowl, then spread out across the prepared tray. Bake for 10–15 minutes, or until aromatic and the coconut is golden brown (be sure to keep an eye on the mixture as it can burn quickly). Remove from the oven and set aside to cool slightly.

Meanwhile, melt your preferred cooking fat in a frying pan over medium heat. Add the apple and fry, stirring and turning often to get good coverage, for 3–4 minutes, or until slightly softened. Stir in the berries and sweetener of choice, if using, and cook, stirring constantly, for 5–6 minutes, or until the berries have broken down and their juices have begun to reduce and thicken.

To serve, spoon half the apple and berry mixture into four wide-mouthed glasses or ramekins then spoon over half the crumble mixture. Repeat with another layer of the apple and berry mixture and crumble.

GOOD TO KNOW: *This recipe can be made in bulk ahead of time — simply whip up a big batch of both elements, store them in the fridge separately and plate it up when it's time to serve.*

HEALTH HACK: *I love cooking with butter as dairy from grass-fed cows is packed with minerals as well as the fat-soluble vitamins A, D, E and K, which can help balance out our hormone levels.*

PEANUT BUTTER CREAM COOKIES

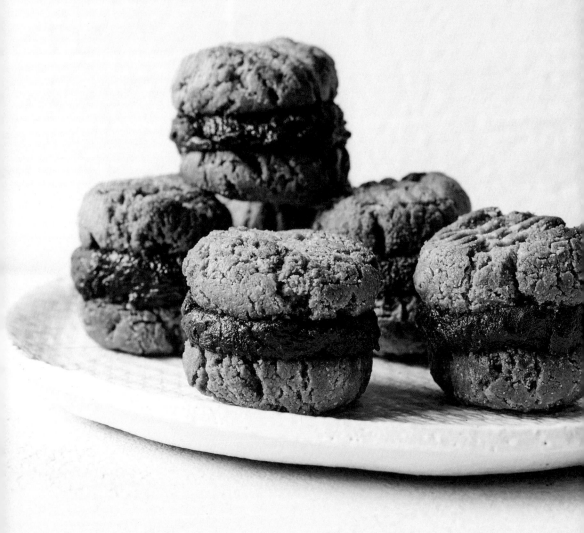

WHEN I WAS A KID THERE WAS A CAFE ON THE WAY HOME THAT SOLD THE MOST DELICIOUS YO-YOS. THEY REALLY WERE AMAZING. HERE, I'VE TAKEN THAT LOVELY MEMORY AND MIXED IT WITH MY LOVE OF PEANUT BUTTER TO BRING YOU THESE PEANUT BUTTER CREAM COOKIES. YOU CAN THANK ME LATER.

MAKES 6

250 g (1 cup) smooth peanut butter
55 g (½ cup) almond meal
2 eggs, beaten
2 tablespoons monk fruit syrup or
   1–2 drops of liquid stevia
1 teaspoon vanilla bean powder
   or extract

PEANUT BUTTER CREAM FILLING

75 g (½ cup) roughly chopped Luke's
   Block of Choc (see page 158)
3 tablespoons canned coconut cream
3 tablespoons smooth peanut butter
1 tablespoon monk fruit syrup or
   ½–1 drop of liquid stevia (optional)

Preheat the oven to 160°C and line a large baking tray with baking paper.

Combine the peanut butter, almond meal, egg, sweetener of choice and vanilla in a bowl and mix well with a wooden spoon to form a dough. Divide the dough into 12 equal-sized pieces, then roll each piece into a ball.

Space the balls out on the prepared tray and gently press with a fork to flatten them (and create that awesome little imprint). Bake for 12–15 minutes, or until lightly golden brown. Remove from the oven and set aside to cool completely.

While the cookies are cooling, make the filling. Melt the chocolate in a small saucepan over low heat, stirring, until thick and creamy. Remove from the heat and leave to cool slightly, then whisk in the coconut cream, peanut butter and sweetener of choice, if using. Remove from the heat and leave for 15–20 minutes to cool and thicken up.

Once the cookies and filling have cooled, spread the filling over the bottoms of six of the cookies. Sandwich with the remaining cookies and you're good to go.

GOOD TO KNOW: *These cookies will keep for up to 7 days in an airtight container in the fridge.*

HEALTH HACK: *If you're following a strict paleo diet, simply swap out the peanut butter here for almond, macadamia or Brazil nut butter instead.*

HEAVENLY HEMP SLAB

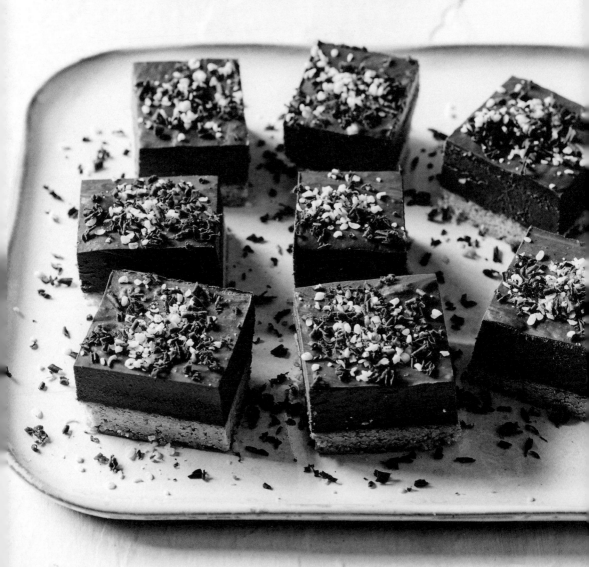

I LOVE TO USE HEMP SEEDS IN MY RECIPES AS THEY BRING SUCH A GREAT NUTTY FLAVOUR AND CRUNCHY TEXTURE TO THE MIX, ALONG WITH SOME AWESOME HEALTH BENEFITS. FOR ANYONE FOLLOWING A LOW-CARB, HEALTHY-FAT APPROACH TO EATING, THEY'RE PRETTY MUCH THE PERFECT INGREDIENT.

MAKES 16 PIECES

BASE
200 g (2 cups) almond meal
85 g (½ cup) hulled hemp seeds
    (hearts)
125 ml (½ cup) coconut oil, grass-fed
    butter or ghee, softened
1 egg
2–4 drops of liquid stevia or
    125 ml (½ cup) monk fruit syrup
pinch of sea salt

FILLING
400 g Luke's Block of Choc
    (see page 158)
500 ml (2 cups) canned
    coconut cream
liquid stevia or monk fruit syrup,
    to taste (optional)

TOPPING
85 g (½ cup) hulled hemp seeds
    (hearts)
50 g Luke's Block of Choc
    (see page 158), shaved

Line a 20 cm square cake tin with baking paper.

For the base, pulse all the ingredients in a food processor or high-speed blender to form a wet dough. Transfer to a bowl and place in the fridge for 10 minutes to firm up.

Once firmed, remove the dough from the fridge and roll it out between two pieces of baking paper into a rough square about 2 cm thick. Turn the tin upside down and press it into the pastry to create the perfect shape for the base, then place your tin on the bench.

Peel the top sheet of baking paper off the pastry. Holding on to the bottom sheet of paper, pick the pastry up and lay it over the base of your tin. Use a sharp knife to trim away any excess pastry so that none goes up the sides of the tin, then transfer it to the fridge to chill for 10–15 minutes.

Preheat the oven to 180°C.

Using a fork, pierce the chilled pastry base a few times, then bake for 25–30 minutes, or until golden brown and crunchy. Remove from the oven and set aside to cool in the tin.

To make the filling, melt the chocolate in a small saucepan over low heat, stirring, until thick and creamy. Remove from the heat and leave to cool slightly, then gradually whisk in the coconut cream until smooth and set aside to thicken. Taste and add your sweetener of choice, if desired. (I always start with 1 tablespoon of syrup and taste before adding more.)

Once cooled, pour the filling over the base, transfer to the fridge and leave for 1–2 hours, or until set.

To serve, cut into 16 squares and sprinkle over the hemp seeds and shaved chocolate to finish.

GOOD TO KNOW: *This slice will keep in an airtight container in the fridge for up to 7 days and can be frozen for up to 3 months.*

HEALTH HACK: *Being rich in healthy fats, high-quality protein and several minerals, hemp seeds may be one of the few superfoods worthy of their reputation. They can now be found in most major supermarkets and health food stores.*

MACADAMIA COCONUT FAT BOMBS

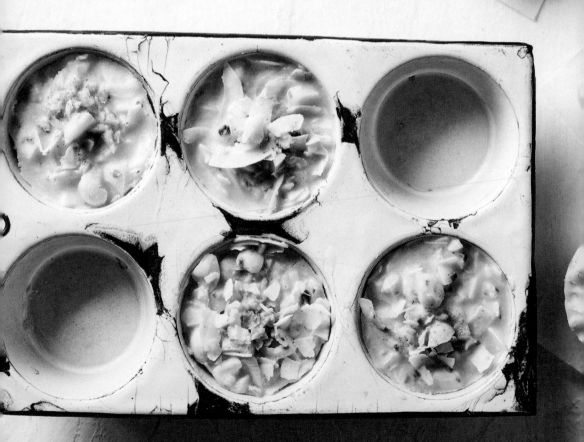

USUALLY MADE FROM A COMBINATION OF INGREDIENTS SUCH AS BUTTER, COCONUT OIL, NUTS AND SEEDS, FAT BOMBS WERE ORIGINALLY DESIGNED FOR THOSE FOLLOWING A STRICT KETOGENIC DIET AS A WAY OF GETTING ENOUGH GOOD FATS. MY VERSION TRANSFORMS THESE INTO BITE-SIZED MORSELS OF DELICIOUSNESS, AND MAKES AN EASY TREAT FOR ANYONE GOING LOW CARB TO FILL UP ON.

MAKES 12

110 g (2 cups) coconut flakes,
  lightly toasted
330 g (2 cups) macadamia nuts,
  toasted and roughly chopped
250 g (1 cup) coconut butter
115 g (½ cup) cacao butter
125 ml (½ cup) coconut oil
2 tablespoons MCT oil
1 teaspoon vanilla bean powder
  or paste
2–4 drops of liquid stevia or
  125 ml (½ cup) monk fruit syrup,
  or to taste
pinch of sea salt

Line a 12-hole muffin tray with paper or silicone cases.

In a dry frying pan over medium heat, toast the coconut and macadamias, tossing them frequently, for 3–4 minutes or until fragrant and just lightly golden brown. Remove from the heat and set aside to cool slightly.

In a saucepan over very low heat, melt the coconut butter, cacao butter and coconut oil. Add the MCT oil, vanilla and sweeter of choice and whisk to combine.

In a large bowl, mix the macadamias and coconut with the creamy choc-coconut mixture.

Spoon the mixture evenly into the prepared muffin tray. Transfer to the fridge and leave for at least 15 minutes to chill and set.

These fat bombs will keep in an airtight container in the fridge for up to 7 days or in the freezer for up to 3 months.

GOOD TO KNOW: *I have chosen to use macadamias here for their incredible health properties, including their wonderful omega-3 to omega-6 ratio, but you can always swap these out for other nuts if you prefer.*

HEALTH HACK: *While MCT oil is great in coffee and smoothies, I have chosen to use it here as I wanted to demonstrate its versatility. As well as being used in treats like this, try drizzling it over salads or adding it to sauces.*

MIXED BERRY MOLTEN LAVA POTS

SERVES 4

coconut oil, for greasing
200 g Luke's Block of Choc
   (see page 158), melted
500 g (2 cups) smooth peanut or
   macadamia butter
250 ml (1 cup) monk fruit syrup,
   maple syrup or coconut nectar
1 teaspoon gluten-free baking powder
pinch of sea salt
2 eggs, beaten
280 g (2 cups) blackberries or
   blueberries, or a mix of both,
   plus extra to serve

Preheat the oven to 170°C and grease four 250 ml (1 cup) ramekins with coconut oil.

Melt the chocolate in a small saucepan over low heat, stirring, until thick and creamy. Remove from the heat and leave to cool slightly, then pour into a mixing bowl. Add the peanut or macadamia butter, sweetener of choice, baking powder and salt and mix well, then add the egg and mix again until well incorporated.

Divide the mixture evenly among the ramekins and spoon a quarter of the berries into the centre of each. Bake for 20–25 minutes, or until the tops are set and slightly cracked but the puddings are still a little wobbly in the centre.

Remove the ramekins from the oven and leave to cool slightly. Served topped with a few extra berries.

GOOD TO KNOW: *If you don't have any ramekins, you can always make these in a greased muffin tray instead. Just be careful when turning the puddings out to serve.*

HEALTH HACK: *The berries in these puddings act as an excellent low-fructose sweetener and do a great job of balancing out the bitterness of the dark chocolate. Plus they're packed with powerful antioxidants that help protect our bodies from cellular damage and degeneration.*

MY VERSION OF THIS SIMPLE SELF-SAUCING PUDDING HAS AN ADDED BURST OF COLOUR AND FRESHNESS FROM THE BERRIES. JUST THE THING ON A COLD WINTER'S NIGHT.

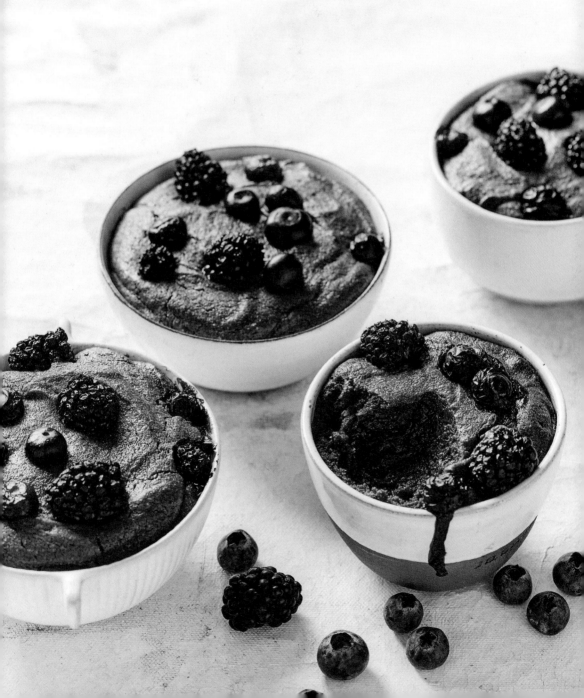

SIMPLE 'SNICKERS' BITES

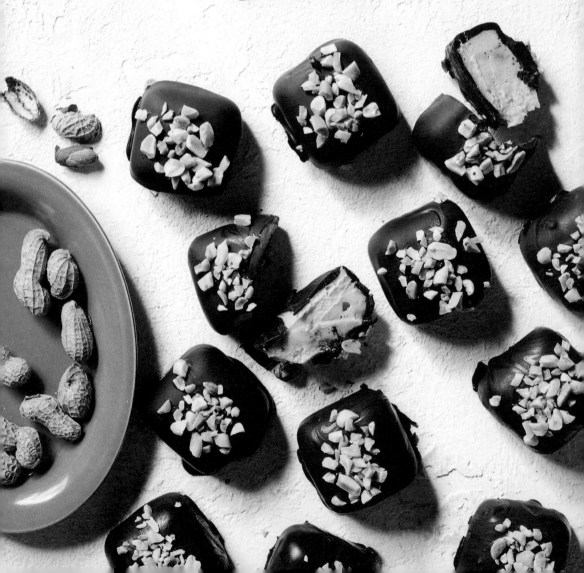

DO YOU REMEMBER THAT OLD SNICKERS COMMERCIAL WITH BETTY WHITE — THE ONE THAT BASICALLY CLAIMED THAT YOU'RE NOT YOU WHEN YOU'RE HUNGRY? WELL I THINK THAT RINGS PRETTY TRUE AND ONCE YOU TRY THESE I CAN ASSURE YOU THAT YOU WON'T BE HUNGRY. IN FACT, I RECKON YOU'LL BE THE HAPPIEST POSSIBLE VERSION OF YOURSELF.

MAKES 12

200 g Luke's Block of Choc
   (see page 158)
80 g (½ cup) peanuts, roughly
   chopped, toasted
sea salt

PEANUT BUTTER FILLING
250 ml (1 cup) canned coconut cream
250 g (1 cup) smooth peanut butter
115 g (½ cup) cacao butter
2–4 drops of liquid stevia or 125 ml
   (½ cup) monk fruit syrup
pinch of sea salt

For the peanut butter filling, place all the ingredients in a saucepan over low heat and melt together, stirring constantly, until nice and runny. Remove from the heat and leave to cool for 10–15 minutes.

Once slightly cooled, pour your mixture into a silicone square ice cube tray and transfer to the freezer to set for a minimum of 1 hour or until completely firm.

When you are ready to assemble the 'Snickers' bites, melt the chocolate in a small saucepan over low heat, stirring as you go, until thick and creamy. Set aside to cool slightly.

Remove one of the frozen peanut fillings from the mould and, using tongs, a spoon or even your fingers, dip it in the melted chocolate. Place on a wire rack and quickly top with the chopped peanuts and a pinch of salt. Repeat with the remaining filling pieces, working quickly before the chocolate completely sets.

Transfer to the fridge for 20 minutes to chill and firm before enjoying. These bites will keep in an airtight container in the fridge for up to 7 days or in the freezer for up to 3 months.

GOOD TO KNOW: *For a thicker chocolate coating, re-freeze the bites after coating with the chocolate (and before sprinkling over the peanuts and salt). Leave to set completely, then coat again before applying the toppings as before.*

HEALTH HACK: *Not only is cocoa butter packed with healthy omega-3s, it also contains a big old dose of phytosterols — plant compounds that can help to reduce bad cholesterol — making it one of the best fats on the block for those following a low-carb diet.*

FURTHER READING

INTERMITTENT FASTING

The benefits of intermittent fasting

Collier, R, 'Intermittent fasting: the science of going without', *Canadian Medical Association Journal*, 2013, vol. 185, no. 9, pp. 363–64.

Fung, J, *The Complete Guide to Fasting*, Victory Belt, 2016.

Heilbronn, LK et al., 'Alternate-day fasting in non-obese subjects: effects on body weight, body composition, and energy metabolism', *The American Journal of Clinical Nutrition*, 2005, vol. 81, no. 1, pp. 69–73.

Johnstone, AM et al., 'Effects of a high-protein ketogenic diet on hunger, appetite, and weight loss in obese men feeding ad libitum', *The American Journal of Clinical Nutrition*, 2008, vol. 87, no. 1, pp. 44–55.

Mattson, MP et al., 'Meal frequency and timing in health and disease', *Proceedings of the Nation-al Academy of Sciences*, 2014, vol. 111, no. 47, pp. 16647–53.

Patterson, RE et al., 'Intermittent fasting and human metabolic health', *Journal of the Academy of Nutrition and Dietetics*, 2015, vol. 115, no. 8, pp. 1203–1212.

Fasting for longer life span

Rose, C, 'Longer daily fasting times improve health and longevity in mice', *National Institute on Ageing*, 6 September 2018, https://www.nia.nih.gov/news/longer-daily-fasting-times-improve-health-and-longevity-mice.

Potential impact on cancer

Cleary, MP & Grossmann, ME, 'The manner in which calories are restricted impacts mammary tumor cancer prevention', *Journal of Carcinogenesis*, 2011, vol. 10, no. 21.

Marinac, CR et al., 'Prolonged Nightly Fasting and Breast Cancer Prognosis' *JAMA Oncology*, 2016, vol. 2, no. 8, pp. 1049–1055.

Potential impact on Alzheimer's and Parkinson's

Duan, W et. al., 'Brain-derived neurotrophic factor mediates an excitoprotective effect of dietary restriction in mice', *Journal of Neurochemistry*, 2001, issue 76, pp. 619–626.

Fasting and gut health

Rong, ZH et al., 'Effect of intermittent fasting on physiology and gut microbiota in presenium rats', *Journal of Southern Medical University*, 2016, vol. 37, issue 4, pp. 423–430, ncbi.nlm.nih.gov/pubmed/28446391

LOW-CARBOHYDRATE DIETS

Benefits of low-carb and keto diets

Adam-Perrot, A et al., 'Low-carbohydrate diets: nutritional and physiological aspects', *Obesity Reviews*, 2006, vol. 7, no. 1, pp. 49-58.

Gedgaudas, N, *Primal Fat Burner: Live Longer, Slow Aging, Super-power your brain, and Save Your Life with a High-fat, Low-carb Paleo Diet*, Atria Books, 2017.

Newman, JC et al., 'Ketogenic diet reduces midlife mortality and improves memory in aging mice', *Cell Metabolism*, 2017, vol. 26, no. 3, pp. 547–57.

Paoli, A et al., 'Beyond weight loss: a review of the therapeutic uses of very-low-carbohydrate (ketogenic) diets', *European Journal of Clinical Nutrition*, 2013, vol. 67, no. 8, pp. 789–96.

Low-carb diets and weight loss

Bueno, NB et al., 'Very-low-carbohydrate ketogenic diet v. low-fat diet for long-term weight loss: a meta-analysis of randomised controlled trials', *British Journal of Nutrition*, 2013, vol. 110, no. 7, pp. 1178–87.

Westman, EC, 'Low carbohydrate nutrition and metabolism', *American Journal of Clinical Nutrition*, 2007, vol. 86, no. 2, pp. 276–84.

CARBOHYDRATES

Human history and carbohydrate consumption

Eaton, SB, 'The ancestral human diet: what was it and should it be a paradigm for contemporary nutrition?', *The Proceedings of the Nutrition Society*, 2006, vol. 65, no. 1, pp. 1–6.

The effects of eating grains

Davis, W, *Wheat Belly: The effortless health and weight-loss solution*, Harper Thorsons, 2015.

Fung, J, *The Obesity Code*, Scribe, 2016.

Mercola, J, 'Eating grains can 'tear holes' in your gut', Mercola, 21 January 2012, articles.mercola.com/sites/articles/archive/2012/01/21/grains-causing-gut-leaks.aspx.

FATS

Why fat is your brain's best friend

Muldoon, MF et al., 'Long-chain omega-3 fatty acids and optimization of cognitive performance', *Military Medicine*, 2014, vol. 179, suppl. 11, pp. 95–105.

Omega fatty acids

Simopoulos, A, 'The importance of the ratio of omega-6/omega-3 essential fatty acids', *Biomedicine and Pharmacotherapy*, 2002, vol. 56, no. 8, pp. 365–79.

Fats and gut health

Zhang, M and Yang, XJ, 'Effects of a high fat diet on intestinal microbiota and gastrointestinal dis-eases', *World Journal of Gastroenterology*, 2016, vol. 22, no. 40, pp. 8905–909.

The benefits of eating grass-fed butter

Fallon, S and Enig, M, *Nourishing Traditions: The Cookbook That Challenges Politically Correct Nutrition and the Diet Dictocrats*, 2003, 2nd edn., pp. 15.

PROTEINS

How protein keeps you satisfied for longer

Chambers, L et al., 'Optimising foods for satiety', *Trends in Food Science and Technology*, 2015, vol. 41, no. 2, pp. 149–60.

Lemon, WR, 'Dietary protein requirements in athletes', *Journal of Nutritional Biochemistry*, 1997, vol. 8, no. 2, pp. 52–60.

CONVERSION CHARTS

Measuring cups and spoons may vary slightly from one country to another, but the difference is generally not enough to affect a recipe. All cup and spoon measures are level.

One Australian metric measuring cup holds 250 ml (8 fl oz), one Australian tablespoon holds 20 ml (4 teaspoons) and one Australian metric teaspoon holds 5 ml. North America, New Zealand and the UK use a 15 ml (3-teaspoon) tablespoon.

LENGTH

METRIC	IMPERIAL
3 mm	⅛ inch
6 mm	¼ inch
1 cm	½ inch
2.5 cm	1 inch
5 cm	2 inches
18 cm	7 inches
20 cm	8 inches
23 cm	9 inches
25 cm	10 inches
30 cm	12 inches

LIQUID MEASURES

ONE AMERICAN PINT	ONE IMPERIAL PINT
500 ml (16 fl oz)	600 ml (20 fl oz)

CUP	METRIC	IMPERIAL
⅛ cup	30 ml	1 fl oz
¼ cup	60 ml	2 fl oz
⅓ cup	80 ml	2½ fl oz
½ cup	125 ml	4 fl oz
⅔ cup	160 ml	5 fl oz
¾ cup	180 ml	6 fl oz
1 cup	250 ml	8 fl oz
2 cups	500 ml	16 fl oz
2¼ cups	560 ml	20 fl oz
4 cups	1 litre	32 fl oz

DRY MEASURES

The most accurate way to measure dry ingredients is to weigh them. However, if using a cup, add the ingredient loosely to the cup and level with a knife; don't compact the ingredient unless the recipe requests 'firmly packed'.

METRIC	IMPERIAL
15 g	½ oz
30 g	1 oz
60 g	2 oz
125 g	4 oz (¼ lb)
185 g	6 oz
250 g	8 oz (½ lb)
375 g	12 oz (¾ lb)
500 g	16 oz (1 lb)
1 kg	32 oz (2 lb)

OVEN TEMPERATURES

CELSIUS	FAHRENHEIT	CELSIUS	GAS MARK
100°C	200°F	110°C	¼
120°C	250°F	130°C	½
150°C	300°F	140°C	1
160°C	325°F	150°C	2
180°C	350°F	170°C	3
200°C	400°F	180°C	4
220°C	425°F	190°C	5
		200°C	6
		220°C	7
		230°C	8
		240°C	9
		250°C	10

THANK YOU

A big delightful thanks to Mary Small, the most wonderful publisher I could ask for, who helps make my dreams come true with each book I get to share with the world. With your backing, belief and unwavering support in all things delicious, I will be singing at the carols in no time.

To Jane Winning, Lucy Heaver and Ashley Carr, I adore working with you guys to bring my books to life. You are so warm and generous with your support, both on set and in the months and months of planning and preparation to bring everything together.

To Mark Roper, Lee Blaylock, Emma Warren and Sarah Watson, it's strange to think that what we do together is work. From Mark's epic shots and Lee's undeniable styling talent, to Emma and Sarah's amazing magic in the kitchen, working with you all is just brilliant. You're the absolute dream team and to me you are family.

To the PR queens Charlotte Ree and Allie Schotte, it's all well and good creating this book, but without your expertise and passion, it wouldn't reach the hands, eyes and kitchens it is much needed in. Thanks for shouting from the rooftops and helping my message be heard far and wide.

Writing and shooting the book is one thing, but without Simon Davis's ingenious editing and Kirby Armstrong's spectacular design we wouldn't have much to show the world. You guys really tie this thing together with a delightful bow.

To my beautiful loved ones, my nearest and dearest close circle in my life. You clap for me in my ups and support me in my downs. You lift me when I need a boost and carry me when I need a rest. Thank you. None of this would be possible without your support, love and belief.

And to my readers: those who have followed me from day one and those who I am meeting right now for the first time. Eleven books is no easy feat and it would never have been possible without your support and backing.

Thank you xx

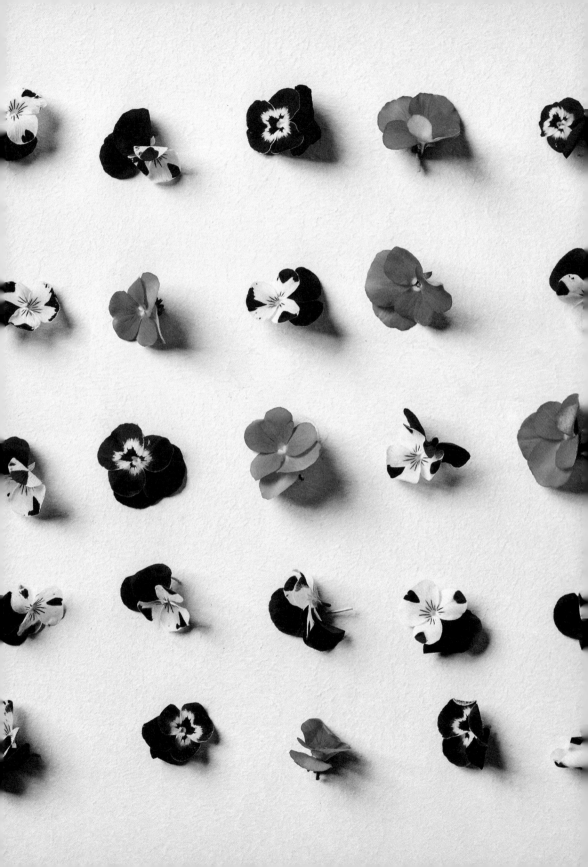

INDEX

A Plum book

First published in 2020 by
Pan Macmillan Australia Pty Limited
Level 25, 1 Market Street,
Sydney, NSW 2000, Australia

Level 3, 112 Wellington Parade,
East Melbourne, Victoria 3002, Australia

Text copyright © Luke Hines 2020
Photography Mark Roper copyright © Pan Macmillan 2020
Design Kirby Armstrong copyright © Pan Macmillan 2020

The moral right of the author has been asserted.

Design and typesetting by Kirby Armstrong
Editing by Simon Davis
Index by Helena Holmgren
Photography by Mark Roper
Prop and food styling by Lee Blaylock
Food preparation by Emma Warren and Sarah Watson
Colour reproduction by Splitting Image Colour Studio
Printed and bound in China by Imago Printing International Limited

A CIP catalogue record for this book is available from the National Library of Australia.

We advise that the information contained in this book does not negate personal responsibility on the
part of the reader for their own health and safety. It is recommended that individually tailored advice
is sought from your healthcare or medical professional. The publishers and their respective employees,
agents and authors are not liable for injuries or damage occasioned to any person as a result of
reading or following the information contained in this book.

10 9 8 7 6 5 4 3 2 1

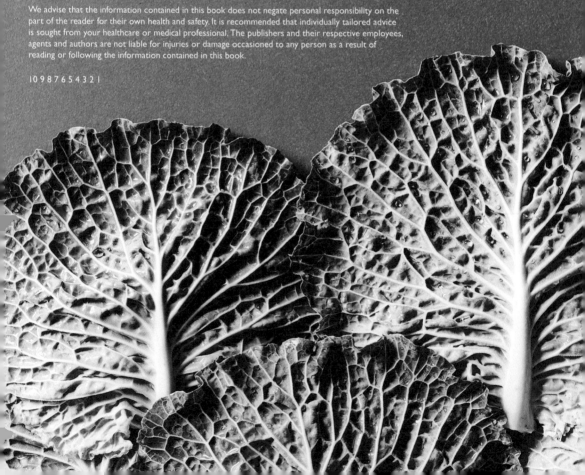